MORAL
MATTERS

Ethical Issues in Medicine and the Life Sciences

ARTHUR CAPLAN

Director, Center for Bioethics
Trustee Professor of Bioethics
University of Pennsylvania

John Wiley & Sons, Inc.
New York / Chichester / Brisbane / Toronto / Singapore

FOREWORD

to

Moral Matters: Ethical Issues in Medicine and the Life Sciences

by Arthur Caplan, PhD

Morality, ethics and law are three of the predominant elements of our culture. They are fundamental controllers of human behavior. Morality is often referred to as an intensely personal feeling, as variable as are individuals; ethics is frequently considered a societal controller that may be standardized and endorsed by various groups; law is public, codified, written, stylized and accompanied by formal sanctions, if transgressed. All are products and expressions of specific cultures.

I consider these three controllers to constitute a hierarchy at the top of which is personal morality. If morality were of sufficient strengths and ubiquity, there would be no need for either societal ethics or public law. Ethics is intermediate in this hierarchy but again, with morality, would be sufficient as controllers of human behavior in a given culture if of adequate power and penetration. The mere existence of examples of the controller lowest in the hierarchy, public law, documents failure of the two higher controllers in those specific areas of societal responsibility.

As our society has evolved, one could easily make the case that personal morality has been declining rapidly, perhaps closely tied to the declining influence of personal and organized religion. So it is not surprising, and is even predictable, that as Controller #1 (morality) declined, Controllers #2 (ethics) and #3 (law) would escalate. And indeed they have.

And that's what this book is all about. Arthur Caplan is in everyone's top 5 list of gurus in the American ethics mafia. Very quick of lip, wit and pen, Dr. Caplan has been, and continues to be, a frequent speaker and commentator and a prolific writer on the toughest medical ethics issues of our time. Soundly grounded in history, philosophy and religion, and always willing to express a strong and clear opinion on even the most vexing individual ethical conundra, Art Caplan is the ideal person to write such a comprehensive collection of essays as one finds in this book. Some of the nearly 100 pieces are new; others have been collected together from recently published works.

Organized into ten realistic chapter headings, they will be perceived as fresh by virtually all readers, both because of the limited distribution of the primary source newspaper where many first appeared and because of author Caplan's own unique style of taking on topical events as they occur, often from breaking news, and analyzing and dissecting them with tart erudition.

Here you find the author's slant on key medical ethical issues of this decade; abortion (medical and surgical), test tube babies, waste of resources, euthanasia, AIDS, violence, homosexuality, gene scares, nicotine and other drugs, diets, lying, and fraud in research, among others.

Short, pithy, topical, timely, stimulating quick reads for a general public audience.

Read, enjoy, disagree and think.

George D. Lundberg, MD
Editor, *The Journal of the American Medical Association*

PREFACE

The essays included in this book began their lives as newspaper columns. Nearly all of them first appeared in the *St. Paul Pioneer Press*, a newspaper based in St. Paul, Minnesota.

Many of my colleagues in academia occasionally express surprise at the fact that I write a column in a medium-size newspaper in a small city. Some, naive about the economics of the newspaper industry, assume the motive must be money. But, there are few occupations in life that pay more paltry fees than being a part-time columnist. Others assume the motive must be egotistical. They are partly correct.

There is a quiet pleasure to be found in seeing your name set in type at the end of a column each week. But, that pleasure only lasts until you have to endure the scrutiny of your readers at what appears in the space. You do need an ego to continue writing columns on controversial subjects, but my experience is that ego helps soften the slings and arrows of critics more than being something which is fed, stroked or inflated by writing columns.

There were two other reasons I decided to write a bioethics column for more than four years. Writing a column lets you stay ahead, if you want to, of developments in medicine and the sciences. Much of bioethics is reactive. Events take place in medicine or the life sciences and those interested in their ethical implications or consequences must react. A column provides a tool that can be proactive. Sometimes, those who are on the receiving end of that proactivity would prefer continued anonymity until they are ready to go public with their work. But, on the whole, ethics is better done before rather than after the fact.

My other reason for writing a column is that it provides a way to talk directly to prospective and actual patients. Bioethics is very much an academic enterprise. The research and teaching of the field take place in large, technologically advanced hospitals and clinics. The tone and content of much of bioethics reflects this fact. Those in bioethics spend much of their time talking to those who provide care or administer the health care system. A column in a newspaper permits some conversation and dialogue to take place outside these circles.

Despite the depressed feelings one has to endure either when the events of the week elicit no musings worthy of print, or the muse itself gets laryngitis, I feel very privileged to have had the chance to write about bioethics for a general audience. I would like to thank Deborah Howell, who was the editor of the *St. Paul Pioneer Press* and who is now with *Newhouse Newspapers* in Washington, D.C., for having the guts to go with weekly columns on bioethics long enough for me to begin to figure out how to do them. I would also like to thank Ken Doctor, Ron Clark, and the other editors at the *Pioneer Press* whom I have had the pleasure of working with over the years for their patience, good humor and insightful suggestions. Not once did they ever make me change a word but they often made it clear to me why I ought to do so.

I would also like to thank Sally Cheney and Erica S. Liu for getting this book done expeditiously.

I must also thank my family, my wife Jane and my son Zach, for their role in making the columns collected in this book possible. Jane is my toughest and most perceptive sounding board. Zach is my most honest critic.

There are a lot of people who write books about ethics in the hope that their readers will accept what they have to say. I am not one of them. I hope no one who reads the essays in this book takes them at face value. This book is supposed to make you think. If you are willing to spend your time reading them closely, so closely that you find flaws and mistakes in my reasoning, then they are serving their purpose. There are many better arguments that can be made about every one of the subjects in this book. So go to it.

Arthur Caplan

INTRODUCTION

To help you get started in reading this book, consider the following four statements. First, ethics is all a matter of opinion. Second, decisions about ethics ought to be left in the hands of ethics experts. Third, ethics cannot possibly keep up with developments in medicine and science. And, finally, those who do ethics never say what they think is right or wrong. I think each of these statements is false. And the reasons why they are false should supply you with some of the tools you will need to read the various essays that make up this book.

It is true, but only in a trivial sense, that morality is a matter of opinion. Much of what passes for moral conversation in our society is simply people venting their feelings about one issue or another. But, while this sort of "shoot from the hip" moral opinionating might often be confused for an ethical argument, it should not be.

Ethics is not the same as morals. Morality refers to what people ordinarily believe about right and wrong, good and bad, virtue and vice. They have these beliefs as a result of attending church, belonging to various civic organizations, watching television programs, listening to their parents, and for innumerable other sociological and cultural reasons. The fact that you learned your morals at your mother's knee does not make your beliefs false or erroneous. But to do ethics you must be willing to do more than simply share your opinions about what is right or wrong, good or bad. You must be prepared to back up your opinions with an argument.

But not any argument will do. You will need to find reasons and evidence that people who do not share your upbringing, your culture, your educational and religious experiences, find understandable and persuasive. Your argument must be able to stand up to challenge on either factual or logical grounds. And your argument must be consistent with arguments you might make about other related issues.

The essays in each chapter of this book are brimming with opinions—nearly all of them mine. But, each essay presents an argument, or sometimes more than one, in support of these opinions. As you read through the book you will find opinions expressed with which you do agree and don't agree. However, your task is not simply to find out how much your opinion and mine overlap or diverge. Your task is to see whether you find the arguments given in support of a position persuasive or not, even if you agree. It is in the scrutiny of the arguments given in support of an opinion that ethics is to be found.

Nor should you be put off from trying to critically read this book by the worry that the experts know better than you. People who study ethics, whether they be theologians, philosophers, or jurists do gain expertise in the identification of moral issues, the classification of moral problems, and in the ways in which arguments from various religious, philosophical, legal and literary traditions can be brought to bear to support or attack a particular position.

But, the experts' views should serve only as a guide to you in forming your own opinions. Most of the issues examined in this book consist of moral problems that could happen to anyone. You or your friend could well face many of the quandaries or dilemmas presented in these pages. You and no one else will have to decide what to do, whether it be in your own home or in the voting booth. In the end, while you may want to hear what those with ethical expertise think about an issue, you must decide for yourself what you believe, what sort of person you wish to be and how to act. Honing your ethical skills by thinking critically about these essays will help you think more clearly about the moral challenges and ethical puzzles that will inevitably arise in your own life where you are the expert.

The idea that ethics cannot keep up with all the many problems and issues that medicine and science spin off as they progress has almost become a truism in our society. That is too bad because nothing could be further from the truth.

Medicine and science do move quickly. And the tools of ethics, a knowledge of the facts, the values and principles of the various moral traditions, both religious and secular, do not. Yet, the tools of ethical argument can meet the challenge of allowing us to deliberate about the merits and challenges of medical and scientific achievements. The only reason medicine and science can leap ahead of our ethics is if we choose to allow that to happen.

Medicine and science are social enterprises. They require huge societal resources and support. Take them away and the pace of medicine and science slows to a crawl. The only obstacles to our thinking through the ethical issues raised by advances in medicine and science is a fear that consensus cannot emerge from complexity or a worry that the answer that is reached may be wrong. But, neither of these concerns shows that ethics cannot keep up. They merely show that the task is sometimes hard and that ethics, like medicine and science, sometimes arrives at the wrong answers.

By the time you are finished reading this book, you will certainly be aware that the last of the four statements I mentioned above, those who study or teach ethics will not give their own views, is surely false. A friend of mine once joked that there is no such thing as an ethicist with one hand because they are always saying, "well, on the one hand, but on the other." The joke is a good one but it rests on a misconception.

Most moral philosophers and theologians that I know are actually quite willing to offer their views as to what is wrong, right, good, sinful or virtuous. By the time you are finished reading this book you will have a pretty good idea of where I stand on many of the topics presented. That is as it should be. In an ethical discussion, you should let others know where you stand. But, the crucial test of whether that is a good place to be is whether your position can hold up to their questions, doubts, criticisms and corrections. And no less holds true for the opinions ventured within these covers.

Arthur Caplan

CONTENTS

CHAPTER 1
ABORTION, CONTRACEPTION, SEXUALITY AND THE FAMILY

Norplant Drug Gives Birth to New Worries

Let me be clear at the outset: There should be no obstacles in the path of women who want to use the new implantable contraceptive drug, Norplant—the most convenient and reliable birth-control agent ever. For women who can't afford it, the government should pay.

But because Norplant is so easy to use, requiring nothing more than the surgical implantation of six matchstick-size implants under the skin, it is irresistibly tempting to those who see the control of women's reproductive behavior as the cure to many of society's ills.

A California judge already has punished a woman by sentencing her to have Norplant put in her arm. Various goofball legislative proposals have been floated in Kansas and other states, and whispered in Congress, to make using Norplant a condition for receiving welfare benefits.

Government-mandated birth control for competent women—even women who are prostitutes, drug addicts, child abusers or welfare cheats—is a terrible idea. The state should not have the authority to manipulate reproduction as punishment or for social engineering.

The argument that the government should not be allowed to coerce women's reproductive choices sounds quaint when our Supreme Court, in its abominable Rust vs. Sullivan decision, allows the government to gag doctors who work in publicly funded clinics. But consider the situation regarding Norplant in Indonesia, if you think government control over reproductive choices is not a bad idea.

Indonesia is a leader in the battle on overpopulation. "Overpopulation" is itself a fighting word, since some believe that Earth is capable of supporting a lot more humans than currently reside here—but if ever there were a nation that qualifies as overpopulated, Indonesia is it. One hundred and ninety million people occupy this Southeast Asian island nation, the fifth most populous on Earth.

Despite its high population, Indonesia has made remarkable strides in controlling its population. Margot Cohen, writing in the April, 1991 issue of the *Far*

Eastern Review, notes that population growth fell from 2.32 percent per year in the 1970s to 1.97 percent per year in the 1980s.

This decrease was the result of a vigorous government program to encourage families to have no more than two children. But the availability of Norplant seems to be causing a shift in Indonesian policy from encouragement to coercion.

Since 1987, according to Cohen, the Indonesian government has been conducting "safaris" in which teams of government officials, sometimes including military personnel, descend on villages to recruit women to use Norplant.

These teams are given strict quotas as to the numbers of women they are expected to recruit to get the drug put in their arms. Those on the safaris are trained to put Norplant in—but apparently less well-trained to take it out. Nor are they always careful to make sure that the women who get implants are not pregnant, which could imperil their fetuses.

Under the pressure of quotas, the safari teams do not always take the time to get full, informed consent from women. It is not hard to imagine the pressure felt by women in these villages in the face of the government's Norplant safari blitzes. And the government itself feels the unyielding pressure an exploding population puts on the social fabric of Indonesia. But that is precisely why we must continue to insist on choice and not coercion where Norplant is concerned.

The choice of whether to reproduce must remain inviolate, lest the state wind up being the sole arbiter of who may parent and who may not.

Birth Control an Ancient Issue, Historians' Research Finds

Population control was not much in evidence at the Earth Summit in Rio. Even though the biggest threat to our environment comes from the ever-expanding number of people that occupy this planet, family planning was left off the agenda.

One reason it is hard to even talk about contraception is that it seems as if ethics and public policy cannot keep up with medical breakthroughs, such as "the pill" or Norplant. But, a fascinating article in the June, 1992 issue of the *American Scientist* should make us think twice about the supposition that birth control is a modern issue.

In the article, two historians, John M. Riddle of North Carolina State and J. Worth Estes of Boston University, argue that both in ancient and medieval times, women used certain plants and herbs to control their reproduction.

Their article shows that the extensive use of birth control throughout history has been lost, distorted or suppressed. The Egyptians, Greeks, Romans, and early Christians were quite willing to practice what the world leaders in Rio are afraid to even talk about.

According to Riddle and Estes, women in ancient times were very familiar with the contraceptive properties of various plants. One port city, Cyrene in North Africa, had birth control as its primary industry.

As early as the 6th century B.C., the Cyrenians were cultivating and exporting huge quantities of silphium, a kind of giant fennel plant. These plants were shipped all over the ancient world. Silphium seeds were crushed and turned into what one ancient writer called "Cyrenaic juice," which women took to prevent contraception. The trade in silphium was so brisk that the plant became a symbol of the city, showing up on most Cyrenian coins.

In the early and middle ages, a host of plants were made into potions or drinks to prevent contraception or cause menstruation. Riddle and Estes say that early doctors from Roman times through the Middle Ages prescribed plants such as wormwood, artemisia, resin from myrrh, pennyroyal, Queen Anne's lace, squirting cucumber and rue to reduce fertility.

Did these early contraceptives work? Riddle and Estes admit that it is impossible to know with certainty. Many ancient historians and scholars describe these herbal potions as effective. And population growth did not seem to be as much of a problem as it should have been in ancient times.

Demographic records from the Roman Empire and the early Middle Ages show there were periodic declines in the populations in Europe and the Mediterranean that cannot be linked to wars or epidemics. It is possible that these unexplained declines were a result of the widespread use of herbal contraceptives.

There are also some recent scientific studies indicating that some of the plants used by the ancients to control fertility do have the capacity to affect female hormones.

Mice given daily doses of extract from the squirting cucumber failed to ovulate. And pulegone, a chemical ingredient of pennyroyal, has been shown capable of inducing abortions in animals and human beings. Seeds from Queen Anne's lace have been shown to inhibit embryo implantation in rats. In fact, women in such disparate places as rural North Carolina and India still chew Queen Anne's lace seeds to reduce their fertility.

If various plants were widely used with some effect by ancient peoples to control their fertility, why is this not widely known? If human beings have long controlled their fertility using contraceptives or drugs that cause menstruation, should this fact be a part of our current debate about population control?

There are probably many reasons why ancient contraceptive practices have been lost. Record keeping in ancient times was poor and wars led to the destruction and loss of much information on ancient medical practices. The rise of Christianity and Islam seems to have led to the repression of knowledge about ancient and medieval birth control practices.

The fact that women controlled the use of plants for contraception may have kept this information outside the mainstream of male-dominated science and medicine.

And, modern medicine's skepticism about folk medicine may have led researchers to ignore promising leads or suggestive lay practices with respect to the control of fertility.

Our female forebears apparently knew a thing or two about birth control. The reason why we cannot be sure exactly what they knew is the same as one that accounts for our continued reluctance to talk about population control and family planning today—morality, medicine and sex make for a highly combustible mix.

Don't Let State Get a Foothold in Reproduction

Some provinces in the People's Republic of China have begun prohibiting people who are mentally retarded, born with severe physical impairments or suffer from mental illness from getting married unless they are sterilized. Should someone with one of these problems get pregnant, an abortion is mandatory.

Prime Minister Li Peng supports these newly enacted laws. He told a parliamentary committee that "mentally retarded people give birth to idiots." An editorial in the quasi-official government newspaper *Peasants Daily* opined that a national law requiring sterilization and mandatory abortion for the retarded was overdue since "idiots produce idiots."

These sentiments are not unique to China. Only a few years ago, the prime minister of Singapore proposed banning marriage among those with low IQs and instituted a system of cash payments to encourage more offspring from those thought to be of exceptional intelligence.

Hitler and his minions were keen enthusiasts for using law to promote coerced sterilization, mandatory abortion and eugenic goals with genocidal results. Even U.S. Supreme Court justices have not been above a kind word for eugenics. Justice Oliver Wendell Holmes foreshadowed Li's thoughts by about six decades when he said, in reference to the constitutionality of a state law requiring forced sterilization of the retarded, "Three generations of idiots is enough."

The usual response to those such as Li, Hitler and Holmes is to point out that eugenics does not work. Most retardation and mental illness are caused by environmental, not genetic factors. The mentally ill, the retarded and the "idiots" are made far more often than they are born.

But what if eugenics did work? What if it were possible to know in advance whether an embryo or fetus would be born with severe intellectual deficiencies? What if your doctor could predict that your fiance, whom you see as Mr. Right, might not be so right given the outcome of the throw of the genetic dice that your marriage would likely produce?

The human genome project, a billion-dollar, taxpayer-funded effort to figure out exactly what messages are encoded in our DNA, will make such predictions possible within a decade or two.

Don't get me wrong. My worries about China's new eugenics laws are not meant to persuade you to urge your representative in Congress to scotch the project. The human genome project ought to be funded and enthusiastically supported.

Decoding our genetic blueprint will revolutionize the way medicine is practiced. Doctors will be able to get beyond treating the symptoms of diseases, such as cystic fibrosis, sickle-cell anemia and juvenile diabetes, and get on with curing the diseases themselves.

But knowledge of human heredity can be put to immoral as well as moral purposes. When we finally learn how to predict retardation and mental illness, let's hope we are not so stupid as to have given government control over reproductive choices.

The burst of sterilization and abortion laws promoted by the current regime in China is a stark reminder that the government that is given the right to decide who can and cannot choose to end a pregnancy or use contraception can quickly become the government that demands that you be sterilized in order to marry.

Abortion Pill May Soon Put
"Operation Rescue" Out of Business

Operation Rescue came to my home town in the summer of 1993. The Twin Cities had the dubious honor of playing host to the militant, nutball fringe of the anti-abortion movement.

There is much to despise about those who target clinics. Those who use harassment as their form of moral argument transform what ought to be the most private and personal decision, whether or not to have a baby, into a public event.

Attempts to shut down abortion clinics by either bombing them or blockading them represent a complete failure of morality. Instead of trying to persuade women that abortion is wrong, the zanies who chain themselves to clinic doors substitute coercion for persuasion.

However, those who think harassment is a reasonable substitute for ethics will soon be out of business. An article on RU 486 in the May 27, 1993 issue of *The New England Journal of Medicine* by a team of French doctors tells why.

RU 486, the so-called abortion pill, has long been available as a non-surgical means of terminating early pregnancies in France, the United Kingdom and Sweden. In its current form the pill must be used in conjunction with another hormone, prostaglandin, which requires an injection by a doctor or nurse.

The French doctors report that they have found a way to administer the prostaglandin in the form of a pill. The pill, misoprostol, which is already sold in drug stores in the United States to help treat stomach disorders, when taken 48 hours after using RU 486, proved in two large studies to be very effective in terminating pregnancies.

The French team concludes their article by noting that the two pill method of abortion "is simpler and potentially allows greater privacy than any other abortion method and it has recently been approved in France."

What does all this research on drugs and pills have to do with Operation Rescue?

Everything. Time and time again we find ourselves wondering about the moral implications of medical progress such as an artificial heart or a test tube baby. Medical progress seems to bring in its wake moral uncertainty. But the possibility of doing abortions without doctors, surgery or specialized clinics shows that sometimes medical progress can solve moral quandaries.

The fact that a woman can end a pregnancy by swallowing two pills forty-eight hours apart at her doctor's office or even in her own home does not make abortion morally right. But, the ability to use pills instead of surgery to end a pregnancy does make abortion a matter of personal, private choice.

For decades our society has been torn apart by deep differences of opinion as to what our laws should say about abortion. But, the controversy only exists as a result of the fact that abortion has been a public act. Up until now, safe abortions required trained specialists working in specially equipped facilities.

But the public nature of abortion is about to change. Whereas pickets and clinic guards once framed the terms of the abortion debate there will soon be nothing more than a woman and a pill.

Operation Rescue and its ilk will soon be history. Abortion is about to become a matter of ethics not politics.

Battles Over Abortion Moving
Into Medical Classrooms

The battle over abortion has taken yet another strange twist. Pro-Choice Resources of Minnesota, a non-profit abortion rights organization, has awarded a $1,500 scholarship to a third-year medical student who is enrolled at the University of Minnesota's medical school.

There is certainly nothing wrong with an organization making money available to financially strapped students. But this scholarship came with a condition. To qualify for the award, recipients must pledge to be willing to perform abortions as one of the services they will provide when they become physicians.

According to officials at Pro-Choice Resources, their scholarship is the first in the country of its kind. The group wants to make sure that in the years to come there will be physicians trained and willing to perform abortions.

While the young woman who received the award this year has not yet decided on her medical specialty, she says she wants to provide comprehensive medical care to women and children and that such care will include first-trimester abortions.

The announcement of the scholarship set off the predictable tantrum so familiar in the abortion debate in this country. Anti-abortion leaders spoke of creating a counter-scholarship fund to educate young physicians about the evil of abortion. Some true zanies talked about creating a Joseph Mengele prize for physicians who perform abortions.

Abortion rights groups all around the United States do have reason for concern about the availability of doctors competent and willing to do abortions. Vast regions of the country have no doctors or clinics willing to do the procedure. In some states, such as North Dakota, there is only a single doctor doing abortions.

According to experts at New York City's Alan Guttmacher Institute, the number of abortion providers, including both individual doctors and clinics, has declined by more than 10 percent in the past five years.

Why the decline?

Some states have enacted legislation that makes it difficult to offer the procedure. Many states and the federal government have restricted funding for women who rely on government programs to pay for the procedure.

The prospect of harassment, picketing and death threats undoubtedly has led some doctors, clinics and hospitals to stop offering abortions. And undoubtedly shifts in medical thinking about the morality of elective abortion played a role.

Pro-Choice Resources hopes that, by funding young doctors who are pro-choice, they can ensure the availability of abortion. But, even if there are students willing to learn and perform abortions, is medicine willing to teach them how?

Fewer doctors are expected to know how to do abortions as part of their medical specialty training. Abortions are not taught in medical school. The procedure is taught after medical school in specialty training. And in the specialty where specialists are most likely to be asked to do abortions, obstetrics and gynecology, training is on the decline.

A 1992 survey by Dr. Trenton McKay of the obstetrics and gynecology department at the University of California, Davis Medical Center, of students in residency programs in obstetrics and gynecology showed that only 12.4 percent of all students are routinely taught how to do first-trimester abortions and only 6.7 percent learn second-trimester abortion procedures. More than 30 percent of all programs do no training in the procedure.

In 1985, the numbers reported for routine training for first- and second-trimester abortion, according to officials at the American College of Obstetrics and gynecologists, were 22.6 percent and 20.6 percent, respectively.

So, in seven years, there has been a precipitous decline of more than half in the number of obstetricians and gynecologists who are required to know how to do abortions.

The battle over abortion usually takes place in very public places: at abortion clinics, in marches on the nation's capital, on the floors of state legislatures and in the nation's courts.

But the battles over abortion are being waged in much more private arenas such as the medical school classroom and the teaching rotation. Ultimately, as Pro-Choice Resources realizes, these battles may be as important as any other in determining what happens to abortion in this country in the future.

Quietly, with Inaction, Court Settles
Central Abortion Issue

It is hard to believe, but the debate about the legal availability of elective abortion in this country is over. The issue that has done more over the past two decades to tear this nation apart than any other came to an end with a whimper, rather than a bang.

The abortion debate's death took place in the U.S. Supreme Court on Nov. 30, 1992. Its passing was so quiet that few people seem to have noticed. But it is over.

Maybe the end of the debate went unnoticed because those who have spent the better parts of their lives engaged in it refuse to believe or are simply incapable of believing that the fight could possibly be over. Fanaticism can make it hard to let go of one's opponent.

Those who oppose elective abortion think that if they redouble their efforts their side can still win absolute victory in the state legislatures, city councils, county boards or in Congress. They are wrong. The legal availability of elective abortion in the first trimester of pregnancy can no longer be removed by either legislative or judicial action.

Those on the choice side think they must struggle on to ensure elective abortion as a fundamental right. They are wrong.

While there are many battles yet to come, they will all be on the periphery. The core issue of the last 20 years of debate—whether women have a constitutional right to elective abortion—has been settled in their favor.

The availability of elective abortion was assured when the Supreme Court refused to hear an appeal of a ruling issued in April, 1992 by the 9th Circuit Court of Appeals in San Francisco.

The territory of Guam enacted a law in 1990 banning elective abortions in all cases except those in which the life of the mother is gravely threatened. The Court of Appeals found this law "clearly unconstitutional." The governor of Guam, who opposes the availability of elective abortion, filed an appeal to the Supreme Court.

Six of the nine judges, including Reagan-Bush appointees O'Connor, Kennedy, Souter and Thomas, after spending weeks considering the case, declined to hear it.

Sometimes a failure to act has greater consequences than acting. When the Supreme Court failed to act, it let the appeals court decision stand. This means that the Supreme Court has now affirmed a constitutional right to elective abortion. Future high courts would be hard-pressed to disregard the message sent by this Supreme Court in letting the Guam decision stand.

It is true that the Supreme Court has indicated that legislators may place restrictions on elective abortions as long as they do not pose an "undue burden." Since no one is exactly sure what an undue burden is, many who oppose the legal availability of abortion will seek to enact laws that can meet this test.

But arguing over which if any restrictions do not pose undue burdens for women seeking abortions is a far cry from bans or prohibitions. Women have a basic constitutional right, dating back to Roe vs. Wade and now cast in stone in the Guam case, to end a pregnancy if their fetus is not viable.

Perhaps the end of the debate came so quietly because most participants realize there is little reason for celebration. As so often is true in war, there are no real winners.

Assuring women the right to abortion acknowledges a right to make a choice fraught with uncertainty, doubt and moral ambiguity. It is a right that women must have but one they should not have to invoke.

Those who have fought so hard to assure women legal control over their bodies and their opponents must now seek common ground to minimize the need for elective abortion.

Abortion, like all other choices made by competent adults about sex and procreation, is and ought to be a matter of morality, not law. The end of the legal debate should occasion the start of a moral dialogue.

Our society has too many unwanted pregnancies and thus too many abortions. We are too tolerant of the blatant exploitation of sex in advertising, television, movies and other forms of entertainment. Our culture encourages sexual relations among children and young people who are not prepared to handle the consequences. Our government and our scientists have not done what they should to develop safe, effective and reliable means of contraception.

Now that the debate is over, we need to redirect the energy from the war over abortion to the search for values, principles and public policies that ensure that elective abortion is a right no one must feel compelled to claim.

Castration of Rapist May Not
Change Will, Only the Way

On March 5, 1992, Steven Allen Butler persuaded a judge in Houston, Texas, to drop a sexual-assault charge against him, provided he undergoes surgical castration.

A lawyer for Butler said later that Butler, apparently at the urging of his family, may be changing his mind about having his testicles removed.

Butler was facing a life sentence for repeatedly raping a 13-year-old girl last year. He previously had been convicted of molesting a 7-year-old. Butler is very bad news.

While in jail awaiting trial, Butler read in a magazine that castration might prevent sex offenders from molesting and raping. The prospect of a long stay in jail did not appeal to him. It had so little appeal that he wrote Judge Michael McSpadden and offered to undergo castration in return for his immediate release from prison and having his record cleared if he stays out of trouble for 10 years.

The judge, who has long favored castration for sexual offenders, jumped at the offer.

He made the wrong choice.

Why should a judge be especially interested in what a convicted child molester and rapist has to say about his preference for punishment? The fact that Butler, a 28-year-old father, was willing to plea-bargain away his ability to procreate does not make castration a good idea.

Simply because a prisoner values freedom more than his testicles is no reason for a judge or anyone else to honor his request. And can Butler really make a voluntary choice with a life sentence staring him in the face?

Life outside prison may seem more attractive to him than life without testicles. But what if he were to decide, after a few years, that he would like to have another child? Could he sue Judge McSpadden and the state of Texas for allowing him to mutilate himself when he was in the coercive environment of a prison?

Doctors should not allow their services to be used by the state to punish criminals. In most nations, performing mutilating, irreversible surgery at the order of the police and judges goes under the name of torture, not medicine.

And there are problems with putting someone like Butler back on the streets. Even in a neutered state, a castrated man is still sometimes capable of sexual intercourse, and Butler most certainly would still be capable of bothering and molesting kids in other despicable ways.

Castration, contrary to the dreams of its many proponents in this nation, does not necessarily change the will, only the way.

Finally, every American should be appalled at the prospect of castration being accepted by the legal system as a punishment. Castration for a rapist today may mean forced sterilization tomorrow for the deviant, the different or those seen as overly fecund. Steven Allen Butler should remain attached to his gonads. He should be forced to remain physically intact for a very long time in a secure jail cell.

Worthiness of Single Parenting at Issue in Frozen-Sperm Legal Case

In October 1991, William Kane committed suicide. But before he died, he deposited seven sperm vials at a Southern California sperm bank.

Kane's girlfriend of many years, 37-year-old Deborah Hecht, wanted custody of the frozen sperm so she could use it to try and have a child. Kane's former wife, Sandra Irwin, with whom he had two children, wanted Kane's sperm destroyed. Judge Edward Ross of Los Angeles County Superior Court decided the fate of the vials.

In resolving the case, Judge Ross grappled with such prickly moral brambles as whether it is fair to a child to be created when a parent has already died; what, if any, restrictions should be placed on those who can use a sperm bank; who can be a parent; and whether human sperm should be treated as property.

Hecht's attorney argued that it is very clear William Kane visited the sperm bank before he took his life so that his girlfriend could bear his child. Kane specified in his will that she should have his sperm. And Kane signed a form at the sperm bank authorizing release of his sperm to Hecht or her doctor.

So it seems fair to assume that Kane really did want Hecht to have the right to use his sperm to have a child.

Kane's ex-wife did not really disagree that Kane wanted his girlfriend to get his sperm. But she wants to protect her children's financial interest in Kane's estate. She asked whether Kane's wishes ought to be respected, given that he was despondent enough to kill himself. Moreover, she contended that a court should know that it is in the best interest of a child to be born with both a mother and a father.

Undoubtedly, it is in a child's best interest to come into this world with a full complement of parents. It would also be great if those parents had lots of money, advanced educations, tons of experience in dealing with children and were loving, caring people. But admitting that certain factors contribute to a child's best interest does not mean that their absence will ruin a child's life.

Despite former Vice President Dan Quayle's overheated efforts to use a fictional TV character to prove the evil of single parenting, children can and do flourish in the care of one adult. If life without a mom or dad is not so bad as to make it cruel for a court to allow for single parents, then there would seem to be little reason for a court to say that single women cannot use sperm banks.

If a woman wants to use a particular donor's sperm, then surely she needs his permission. But Hecht seems to have that. So there is still no reason to prevent Hecht from using Kane's sperm if she wishes to do so.

Nor would it be wise for a court to make rules about who can be a parent. This is a matter for public debate and, ultimately, legislation. A court is a lousy place to decide who can be a mom or a dad.

There are those who might say that the case for allowing Hecht to use her former boyfriend's sperm is cinched by the fact that we ought to treat sperm like any other form of property. If a man wants to will his sperm to his girlfriend or, if you or I want to give our eggs or sperm to some lucky recipient, then we ought to be free to do so, since our reproductive materials belong to us.

But property is not the ideal concept to use to resolve the fate of Kane's sperm. Kane had the right to decide what ought to happen to his sperm. But he did not have the absolute right of property, since sperm is the blueprint for another human being and that being needs its interests considered, as well.

So what should be done with William Kane's sperm? There is no convincing reason to think that being born to one parent is so horrid a fate that the law ought not permit it. Since Kane wanted it made available to his girlfriend, she ought to be allowed to use it if she chooses to do so. And that is how the judge ruled.

Wrongful-Birth Lawsuits are Wrong Solution

When Efser Garrison learned she was pregnant, she decided to have an amniocentesis test done. The 39-year-old Delaware woman knew that her age put her at increased risk of giving birth to a baby with Down syndrome, a genetic disorder that causes mild to profound mental retardation, among other problems.

During amniocentesis, a doctor uses ultrasound to guide a needle through the mother's abdomen into the amniotic sac surrounding the fetus. A small amount of fluid is withdrawn. Fetal cells are isolated from the amniotic fluid and grown in a laboratory dish. Then, these cells are analyzed to see if the fetus has certain birth defects, such as Down syndrome.

It takes three or four weeks to get the test results. Then, if Down syndrome is detected, the only options are to continue the pregnancy or abort it.

Something went wrong in Efser Garrison's amniocentesis, and no test results were available. By the time a second amniocentesis could have been completed, it would have been too late—legally—to abort the fetus. Efser gave birth to a daughter, Hope, who is retarded.

According to a Nov. 26, 1991 article in the *Philadelphia Inquirer*, the Garrisons decided to sue the Medical center of Delaware Inc., which owns Christiana Hospital, where the amniocentesis was performed. They claim the failed test caused them to experience a "wrongful birth." The Garrisons' position is that they would have aborted the pregnancy.

The Garrisons are not alone in saying that had they known that their fetus had Down syndrome, they would have ended the pregnancy. The *Southern Medical Journal* has published a comprehensive study by a team of researchers at the University of South Carolina School of Medicine that sheds light on what most parents do when an amniocentesis reveals that their fetus has Down syndrome.

The researchers looked at 26,950 amniocenteses conducted in 14 hospitals in seven states. There were 168 fetuses with Down syndrome detected. Of these pregnancies, 92 percent were aborted.

The Garrisons are not the first to sue over an unwanted birth. Wrongful-birth cases have been brought in New Jersey, Kansas, New York and many other states. But, neither the increasing number of wrongful-birth lawsuits nor the reality that most families decide against having a child with Down syndrome means that the best way to handle a failed prenatal test is to have parents argue in court that their child should not have been born.

What could be worse than risking having a child learn that his or her parents argued in court that if the doctors and hospital had only done their jobs, he or she would have been aborted? Are we so lawsuit-happy in this country that the best we can do is tell parents such as the Garrisons to go to court and zealously argue that their baby is a wrongful birth?

If ever there were an area of medical practice where adversarial legal haggling is inappropriate, it is over matters of wrongful birth. If a test is botched or a doctor fails to offer a prenatal procedure, parents who want to do so should be able to recover damages under binding arbitration by a panel whose deliberations are closed to the public. Monetary awards should be given only to help provide care and support for the families and their children.

But parents should never be forced to state for the record in a court of law that their son or daughter should not have been born. Wrongful birth is a bad idea whose time should never have come.

Two Children's Cases Explore
Formulas for Family Ties

On the same day in August, two children found themselves at the center of bitter legal disputes about exactly what it is that makes a child and an adult into a family.

Kimberly Mays, a 14-year-old ninth-grader, told a judge in Sarasota, Fla., that she never wanted to see her biological parents again.

A thousand miles away, a 2-1/2-year-old tot known as Jessica was taken screaming and crying from the arms of Jan and Robert DeBoer, the only parents she had ever known. She was driven to an Ann Arbor, Mich., police station. There, in accordance with the instructions of a Michigan judge, she was turned over to her biological parents, Dan and Cara Schmidt.

What role does biology play in defining a family? And why has it played such a different role in the cases of Kimberly Mays and Jessica?

There is no doubt that Kimberly is not the child of the man who has raised her since birth, Bob Mays. She is the biological child of Ernest and Regina Twigg. The Twiggs lost their baby in 1979 when the identification tags on two newborn girls were switched in a hospital in Wauchula, Fla.

Kimberly was, unknowingly, taken home by Barbara and Bob Mays. The Mays' child, whom the Twiggs brought home, was named Arlena. The switch was discovered when, a few years later, Arlena developed a serious heart problem. Blood tests done to diagnose the problem showed that she could not have been the Twiggs' baby.

When Arlena died in 1988, the Twiggs tracked down Bob Mays, whose wife had died of cancer in 1981, and demanded that Kimberly be tested to see if she was their biological child. At first, Mays fought the request in court, but eventually he gave in when the Twiggs said they would not seek custody, only visitation rights. A genetic test proved that Kimberly was the Twiggs' child.

The Twiggs and their seven children did have a few visits with Kimberly, but Mays broke them off late in 1990. When the Twiggs tried to reinstate them, Kimberly found herself in a Florida courtroom pleading with a judge to forbid them to see her anymore.

Kimberly should not have to see the Twiggs again if she does not want to. True, they are her flesh and blood. But she had no contact with them for 14 years and is now old enough to decide if she would like to do so or not.

The only dad she has ever had is Bob Mays. Fourteen years is enough time for love to replace the ties of biology.

Jessica's situation is different. Cara placed her daughter for adoption shortly after giving birth to her on Feb. 8, 1991. The DeBoers planned to adopt her, but Cara, who had initially named the wrong man as the father, changed her mind. She told Dan Schmidt on Feb. 27, 1991 that he was the baby's father. A few days later, Cara and Dan decided to marry and to get their daughter back.

An Iowa court agreed with the Schmidts and voided the adoption process in December 1991. The DeBoers fought the Schmidts' request to return Jessica. They argued before courts in both Iowa and Michigan that it would be in the child's best interest to stay with them, since they were the only parents she had ever known.

But the Iowa courts consistently ruled in favor of the Schmidts. After two years of appeals, the Michigan Supreme Court ruled that the Iowa decisions were binding. The DeBoers then appealed to the U.S. Supreme Court, but the highest court in the land refused to overturn the order to return Jessica to the Schmidts.

Mothers who put their children up for adoption should have a reasonable period of time to change their minds. So should fathers. When Cara let Dan know he was the father, he quickly decided he wanted to keep his child. Jessica had been put up for adoption when all the facts surrounding her birth were not known.

While it is true that the DeBoers acted as her parents nearly from the moment of birth, the fact remains that her mom and dad never agreed to the adoption and fought to have her returned for more than two years.

Parents who want to keep their children must be given a reasonable chance to do so even if it breaks the hearts of others who want nothing more than to become a family.

So, how much time must pass before the love of strangers proves to be more powerful a glue in binding a family together than biology? While we might wish it were otherwise, there is no simple algorithm for resolving such a question.

Fourteen years ought surely to be sufficient for love to nullify biology. Two and a half years may not be if a child's biological parent never is given the chance to make a claim of parenthood, or does not agree to placing a baby for adoption.

What Kimberly and Jessica can teach the rest of us is that both biology and love are necessary to make a family, but that neither alone is enough.

Homosexuality and Science: Good News?

For decades, science and medicine pointed toward psychological causes of homosexuality—distant fathers, smothering mothers, early sexual abuse, etc. But in the past few years, scientists and physicians who have been charmed by the siren song of biology have begun to enter the fray.

While it is certainly laudable that efforts are being made to understand the broad range of factors responsible for such complex behaviors as homosexuality, the moral problem with the recent swing toward nature rather than nurture is that those with the keenest interest in homosexuality keep looking to science for their civil rights.

Remember, not so long ago, the nation was agog over the announcement by a California scientist that he had found tiny differences between the brains of 20 men who had died of AIDS (and were thus presumed to be homosexuals) and a small number of brains obtained from men and women who had expired due to other causes. Many in the gay community expressed relief at the news that science finally had found that the cause of their sexual orientation was in their brains.

Now, researchers from Northwestern and Boston universities have published a paper in the Archives of General Psychiatry in which they announce that male homosexuality has its roots in chromosomes, not upbringing. This study has some real scientific meat in it. But in its wake have come wildly unsubstantiated value statements about homosexuality.

The researchers studied the reported prevalence of homosexuality in a large number of identical and non-identical twin brothers of self-proclaimed gay men. They also looked at the sexual orientation of adopted brothers of gay men. They results they report are noteworthy: 52 percent of the biologically identical twin brothers said they, like their brothers, were gay; 22 percent of the biologically non-identical twins reported being gay; only 11 percent of adopted, genetically unrelated brothers of gay men said they were homosexuals.

The rates of homosexuality among biologically related brothers are higher than would otherwise be expected. So, it would appear that heredity plays an important role in causing homosexuality.

And if so, the authors of the study say, then the case for seeing homosexuality as an illness is weakened. And the authors say that "... a biological explanation is good news for homosexuals and their advocates." Maybe not.

Certainly it is important to encourage and fund studies that examine the causes of sexual orientation and behavior. It is important to understand how we come to be who we are, and understanding the etiology of sexual behavior can provide ideas about what it would take to change.

But suppose science were to find that homosexuality is 100 percent genetic (which no one believes) in origin. Would discrimination against homosexuals end? Would bigots reform their beliefs? No. Those who despise homosexuals would simply advocate the development of prenatal genetic tests so that would-be homosexuals could be nipped in the bud. Homophobes would argue for biological engineering for all homosexuals as soon as possible.

Science provides very little good news or bad news about human nature. It tells us much about how we come to be who we are and what we are up against if we want to be different. But it tells us nothing about whether we should want to change who we are or what way of changing would be best. We have to figure that out for ourselves.

CHAPTER 2
INFERTILITY AND TECHNOLOGICAL REPRODUCTION

Science Forces the Issue: Who Is a Mother?

The torrent of advances in reproductive technology is forcing us to examine one of the most basic concepts in our society—who is a mother?

A group of physicians in Israel says that they have strong evidence that implanting newly created embryos into women seeking *in vitro* fertilization is more effective than using embryos that had been frozen. Their findings are important, if only because there are at least 20,000 frozen embryos currently in storage in the United States and other countries. The Israeli study makes it clear that no doctor who has any choice will want to use a frozen embryo. This creates the obvious questions of who should decide and what should be done with the current reserve of frozen embryos.

Doctors at the University of Southern California reported that five of seven women who had experienced menopause were able to deliver healthy babies as a result of *in vitro* fertilization with eggs from other women.

Not only can medicine come up with techniques like *in vitro* for treating infertility, it is beginning to learn how to extend the boundaries of fertility itself. The day looms when it might not be unusual for a woman in her 50s or even her 60s to become a mother.

A California appellate court judge ruled that Anna Johnson, a woman who had been hired as a surrogate mother, had no parental rights over the child to whom she had given birth. Instead, Mark and Cris Calvert, who supplied the egg and sperm, should be recognized as the parents.

The Calvert case reveals how unprepared our society is to cope with the wonders of reproductive technology. The women who became pregnant after menopause in the USC study knew the women whose eggs they used. In fact, they actually selected them to be egg donors. That means that any one of the women who were egg donors might at any time decide they want to make a claim of parenthood based on supplying the egg to a post-menopausal mom who had a baby as a result.

The ability to muck around with reproduction reveals how little consensus exists in our society about what makes a mother a mother. Are you a mother if you supply the egg from which a baby develops? Or are you a mom if you supply the uterine environment and undergo the risk of delivering a baby into the world? Or, as is the case in adoption, are you a mom if "all you do" is supply the love, pay the bills and serve as a lifetime role model to a baby with whom you have no biological or gestational relationship?

The obvious answer is that biology, pregnancy and child-rearing all constitute motherhood. It is also clear that biology, pregnancy and parenting are each sufficient in themselves to lay claim to motherhood. What is not yet clear is what laws, policies and moral rules can best resolve conflicts about motherhood when biology, pregnancy and child-rearing clash.

No Ethical Stance Could Back
Idea of Fetal Egg Donation

A scientist in Scotland, Roger Gosden of the University of Edinburgh, thinks it is possible to use eggs obtained from aborted fetuses to help infertile women have babies. He believes he can do this by transplanting fetal ovaries.

If so, the transplant would benefit women who cannot make their own eggs, either because they have reached menopause or because they have some disorder or disease that makes their eggs abnormal. Gosden says that he has successfully transplanted fetal ovaries in mice and the he will soon be ready to try the technique using human fetal eggs.

Gosden's announcement was met with a storm of controversy. Some commentators immediately pronounced the idea of using eggs from aborted fetuses ethically repugnant. A group of British legislators said they would quickly draft a law to outlaw such transplants. And the British Medical Association said it would move rapidly to crate a commission to examine the issue.

Others did not find the idea so obviously horrible. Professor John Fletcher, a distinguished theologian who directs the University of Virginia's program in biomedical ethics, argues that we ought not to be too hasty in rejecting Gosden's idea.

Taking eggs from aborted fetuses might seem initially bizarre. But, Fletcher argues, it could help women who cannot now find willing donors from whom to obtain eggs. Moreover, harvesting eggs from fetuses would reduce the number of women who now undergo possibly risky hormonal treatments in order to serve as egg donors.

The benefits of fetal transplants might well outweigh our squeamishness about the source. Some infertility specialists in the United States declared that those who find the idea of mining fetal eggs revolting simply do not understand the anguish of women who desperately want to have a child.

I find none of the arguments in favor of fetal egg harvesting persuasive. Moreover, it is not clear to me that those who think critics should shut up have identified a technique that is really valuable, despite the plight of those who suffer from infertility.

Could fetal ovary transplants really be done? All of the eggs that a woman will ever have in her life are present by the 10th or 11th week of fetal development. So the eggs would appear to be there for harvesting if ovaries can really be transplanted.

But a mouse is not a human being. Human reproduction is notoriously difficult to regulate and control. If it were not so hard, there would not be so many frustrated couples seeking to have children who cannot be helped by current medical techniques.

Little is known about the development of eggs in fetuses or about the environment necessary to allow fetal eggs to develop into babies.

Moreover, despite some optimistic assertions to the effect that fetal ovaries may be less vulnerable to rejection by the recipient's natural immunological defense system, a woman who gets a fetal ovary might reject it unless she takes the same battery of immunosuppressive drugs that all organ transplant recipients must now endure.

Even less is known about the ability of fetal ovaries to function once they are removed from a body. A woman who wanted fetal eggs might have to be present at the abortion clinic and ready for the transplant as soon as an abortion had been performed.

Even if the technical difficulties with fetal ovarian transplants could be overcome, there are still serious ethical minefields confronting those who want to see the surgery tried.

Is it really a good idea to allow sperm, eggs or embryos to be used without the consent of the person to whom they belong? Should the law allow someone to be born without the permission of the parent from whom an egg or sperm is obtained? If parenting without consent is a bad idea, then fetuses would obviously be off-limits for harvesting reproductive tissues.

And would it really be in the best interest of a child to be born from the egg of an aborted fetus? Would the women from whose fetuses fetal eggs are procured have the right to claim custody over any child that is born via a transplant? What would the impact be on a child to learn that your grandmother aborted your mother?

Fetal egg donation is the latest in a series of stunning promissory notes about how science is changing the way babies are made. Just in the past few years, we have watched grandmothers give birth to their own grandchildren, post-menopausal women have babies and the first tentative steps toward the creation of human embryo clones.

Science is challenging our definitions of mother, father, parent and child. Society needs to decide whether morality requires that some of the proposed revisions ought to be rejected.

A Sperm Repository that Is Morally Bankrupt

Nestled on a small street between two commercial banks in the Southern California town of Escondido is one of the weirdest banks in America. No, it is not another crumbling savings and loan. Yes, it is exactly the kind of place that gives California a reputation as the mother lode of world-class zaniness.

It's a sperm bank for breeding superbabies.

The Repository for Germinal Choice is the formal name. You may have heard of this outfit under its colloquial name, the Nobel Prize sperm bank. The assets in this bank consist of sperm frozen in liquid nitrogen. The sperm has been obtained from persons of prominence, achievement and genius who are asked to donate their gametes in the hope that infertile couples will use them to produce improved models of humanity.

The bank claims to have deposits in its fridge from noteworthy scientists, some corporate success stories and at least one Olympic athlete. One hundred babies have been created using sperm from the Repository for Germinal Choice. Couples who want to obtain the sperm must be married and must show themselves to be persons of achievement and ability.

The whole enterprise could be dismissed as yet another example of California goofiness, except for the fact that it is far too morally pernicious. The Repository for Germinal Choice has for the past 10 years been practicing eugenics. The aim of the sperm bank is not to help infertile couples have babies or to screen sperm in order to prevent children from being born with congenital diseases. Its goal is to produce higher quality babies.

The ideology behind the repository is that humankind must encourage those with ability to reproduce and pass on their genes if the human species is to survive. The road to earthly salvation lies in mixing better genes to produce better children.

There are plenty of Americans who are willing to chain themselves to the doors of abortion clinics to prevent what they see as the murder of innocent children. Many others are willing to blockade animal-research facilities to prevent the killing of animals. As far as I know, no one has chained himself or herself in protest to the doors of the Repository for Germinal Choice. Someone should.

The creation of a sperm bank aimed at enhancing the genetic makeup of the human species through breeding people who have achieved "success" rests on a number of mischievous assumptions. The notion that achievement equals only success in business, science or athletics is just plain dingy. The causal link between these sorts of achievements and heredity is weak at best.

The idea that corporate leadership or athletic ability can be passed on through selective breeding rests on a crude view of human inheritance. And the idea that anyone should want, must less be allowed, to create babies with an eye toward their genetic stock is a slur on human difference and diversity.

Ironically, it is precisely the values of tolerance and individuality, so inimical to those who would breed for success, that have allowed this nutball operation to survive for so long.

The repository operates with private money, so it is free to continue to pursue eugenics as its guiding light. And since there are almost no rules governing the operation of sperm banks, couples looking for an early competitive edge for Junior are free to try to create him using the precious bodily fluids of a corporate titan or aging biochemist.

Rumor has it that potential depositors for the bank are found by combing the pages of various popular magazines for the names of persons of ability and achievement. If that doesn't give you the willies, it should.

Perhaps we should not worry too much about the efforts of a few poor souls to fulfill their dreams of a super-race in a California suburb. After all, the Repository for Germinal Choice has not been involved in the creation of all that many babies. It has had relatively few depositors and relatively few customers.

But genetic science is on the move around the world. Every day, scientists are finding out more and more about what it is that makes our genes tick. Within the next 15 years, scientists will have sequenced and mapped all the information in the human genome. As genetic knowledge expands, the prospects for making a serious stab at eugenics will, too. The repository's best years may lie ahead.

Let's hope not. Designing our descendants with an eye only on their potential to achieve is not fair to them, and it insults those of us whose achievements and triumphs will never be celebrated on the cover of a popular magazine.

53-Year-Old's Test-Tube Births
Raise Troubling Questions

A 53-year-old California woman gave birth on Nov. 11, 1992 to twins. Giving birth at 53 is remarkable enough, but even more remarkably, the woman had the babies even though she had lost the ability to make eggs.

Mary Shearing and her 32-year-old husband, Don, created the twins using eggs donated by a woman in her 20s. The eggs were then fertilized using a process known as *in vitro* fertilization.

The eggs were surgically removed from the donor and mixed with Don's sperm in a laboratory dish; some of the resulting embryos were then reimplanted in Mary Shearing's womb, where they became Amy Leigh and Kelly Ann.

I heard about the birth of the twins on TV. The newscaster said that Mary Shearing was the first woman to successfully give birth after menopause to twins.

But the ethical issues raised when a 53-year-old woman uses donated eggs to get pregnant are not so simple. Not because a couple is somehow too "old" to be parents. But because the procedure may be too dangerous for the children who are created in this way.

Mary Shearing and her husband, Don, went public in October about their efforts to have a child. They and their doctors at Martin Luther Hospital held a press conference to a rapt audience of dozens of journalists, at which they announced that Mary was the oldest post-menopausal woman ever to become pregnant.

The media quickly grabbed the story and ran out to find people who didn't think what the Shearings were doing was such a hot idea. Some professional hand-wringers, including me, wondered whether it was a good idea for a 53-year-old woman to face the rigors of pregnancy. Others expressed concern about whether it was fair to bring a baby into the world knowing that the kid would be entering high school about the time mom was applying for Medicare.

Don and Mary Shearing weren't very worried about the age factor. "While it is important," Mary said, "it is not something you run your life by."

Their doctor, David Diaz, noted that Mary was in good health and was very fit, making her chances of having a successful childbirth equal to those of a younger woman.

Lots of couples fell asleep arguing about whether grandmoms ought to have babies. But the birth of the twins ought to remind us that more than adult choices and preferences are involved when technology is used to make a baby.

Mary and Don Shearing's twins arrived three months early. One of the 28-week-old twins weighed 2 pounds, 2 ounces, at birth; the other 2 pounds, 12 ounces. They are very low birth weight, very premature babies. And they are the reason we need to proceed more cautiously in using egg donation and *in vitro* fertilization to permit older women to get pregnant.

Premature babies face some very dismal statistics. About a quarter of all children born at 28 weeks die. Roughly one in 10 have severe bleeding in their brains that can cause retardation and other problems. Thirteen percent have chronic lung failure. Nearly a quarter have significant physical or mental impairment.

Premature babies spend a lot of time in neonatal intensive care. The cost of one day for infant intensive care is $2,500. Bills of $50,000 to $100,000 are not at all uncommon for preemies the size of the Shearing twins.

Extreme preemies also face a 30 percent chance of having to go back to the hospital for a long stay at least once during their first year of life because they get another serious illness.

The technology to rescue extremely premature very low birth weight babies is so new that there is relatively little information on how these kids do as adults.

Families like the Shearings ought to be free to have kids without requiring the permission of the government, ethicists or anyone else. But when it comes to reproductive technologies, it is silly and morally irresponsible to behave as if medical science knows what it is doing when it does not.

There are very real risks when older women get pregnant. These can, however, be explained so a woman can choose what she wants to do. The problem with using egg donation in a menopausal woman is that it poses very real even fatal risks not only to the mom but to her babies. There is a very good chance that older mothers will not be able to carry a pregnancy safely to term.

So not only do we need to consider the health of the mother, but also the legal ambiguities about maternity that arise when donor eggs are used, the downside of having older parents and the real risk that any children who result face a real risk of being born too soon—so soon that they risk death or permanent severe disability.

It seems rude, even cruel to say that a technology that holds out the promise of having a child to a desperate woman or couple ought not to be used because it is too risky. Still, the doctors and couples who want to use this technique must remember that they are experimenting with the lives of children who cannot give their consent.

Tennessee Frozen-Embryo Case
Hits Compulsive Parenthood

The Tennessee Supreme Court issued a ruling in May of 1992 concerning the fate of seven embryos frozen in a liquid nitrogen tank in a Knoxville, Tenn., fertility clinic. The opinion has important implications not only for the fate of the more than 22,000 embryos now frozen at clinics around the nation, but also for the national debate about abortion.

Mary Sue and Junior Lewis Davis were married on April 26, 1980. They wanted kids. Mary Sue got pregnant five times. Each time, unfortunately, she suffered a tubal pregnancy. She could conceive, but the embryos kept getting stuck in her fallopian tubes instead of implanting in her uterus.

Finally, she had to have her tubes removed, leaving her able to make eggs but unable to bear a child.

In 1985 the Davises went through six attempts at *in vitro* fertilization. This is the procedure where eggs are microsurgically removed from a woman's ovaries and placed in a dish along with sperm from her husband or another donor. The embryos can then be surgically placed into the uterus.

The Davises had no luck with *in vitro* fertilization. They decided after their last attempt, in December 1988, that instead of giving up they would freeze the seven embryos that grew in the dish in order to try again at some future time.

But Junior Davis filed for divorce in February 1989. He said that he had known his marriage was falling apart for some time, but had hoped that the birth of a baby might have saved it.

The divorce went through. But, there was one sticking point. Who would get custody of the frozen embryos?

No provision or contract had been made at the fertility clinic as to who would have custody of them in the event of a divorce. In fact, most *in vitro* fertilization programs do not have explicit policies about how to handle frozen embryos when couples divorce, remarry or die. That is why there are tens of thousands suspended in a frozen moral limbo in so many refrigerators in the United States and other countries.

Mary Sue wanted custody of the embryos. She originally said she wanted them so she could try to have a baby. Junior Lewis objected. Mary Sue went to court to obtain sole custody.

The first court to hear the case awarded her custody of the embryos on the ground that the embryos were "human beings" from the moment of fertilization and ought to have the "opportunity ... to be brought to term through implantation."

Junior Lewis appealed that decision. Last year a Tennessee appellate court reversed the trial court, assigning joint custody over the embryos on the grounds that Junior had a "constitutionally protected right not to beget a child" without his consent.

Mary Sue decided to appeal this ruling to the Tennessee Supreme Court. She no longer wanted to use the embryos herself. She wanted to donate them to another childless couple rather than have them destroyed. Junior Lewis remained adamantly opposed, preferring that the embryos be destroyed.

In its ruling, the Tennessee Supreme Court scolded fertility clinics for not making the disposition of unused or unwanted embryos part of the consent process. The court rejected out of hand the view that legal or moral rights begin at conception. It found no legal basis for assigning personhood to an eight-cell embryo or giving an embryo the same legal standing as a child.

Instead, the court held that there is a fundamental right to privacy, in the laws of Tennessee and in the U.S. Constitution, that forbids compelling Mr. Davis to become a parent against his will.

The court concluded that "Mary Sue Davis' interest in donating the embryos is not as significant as the interest Junior Davis has in avoiding parenthood," and forbid the implantation of the seven embryos into any woman unless Mr. Davis agrees.

The finding in this case is especially important because it is the first state supreme court ruling in a custody dispute over frozen embryos. The ruling means that very few of the unwanted or unused embryos now in storage will ever be implanted in anyone uterus, certainly in Tennessee and probably elsewhere.

But the significance of the case goes further. The Tennessee Supreme Court has now dismissed the claim that rights begin at conception. It has also asserted the view that no man should be forced to parent against his will. These two rulings have obvious implications for the future of abortion policy in this country.

Those who favor laws granting a right to life to embryos from the point of their conception can be sure that many courts will reach the same conclusion as the Tennessee Supreme Court—there is no constitutional foundation for assigning rights from the point of conception. The U.S. Supreme Court will find it very difficult in deliberating the fate of Roe vs. Wade to ignore the Davis case.

The Tennessee court has sent a clear message that states do not have a right to compel men to become parents against their will.

Will the nation's highest court try to compel women to do what in Tennessee a man cannot be made to do—have a child against his will?

Determining Fetal Sex May Bring
Both Joy, Grief for Society

Since the first human distinguished pink from blue, one of the mysteries and joys of pregnancy has been waiting to learn the sex of the baby.

Modern reproductive technology is on the verge of making birth a bit less mysterious. It remains to be seen whether, as a result, birth will become any less joyous.

For many years medicine has had the ability to determine the sex of a baby while it is still inside its mother's womb. Ultrasound technology allows doctors to use sound waves to take pictures of the developing fetus. An experienced ultrasound observer can almost always figure out the sex by six or seven months into a pregnancy simply by looking.

Doctors can also tell the sex of a baby before it is born by using tests such as amniocentesis or chorionic villus biopsy. In using these tests, a doctor withdraws a small amount of cells from the tissues and fluids that surround the fetus and then looks in a microscope to see if there is an X or a Y chromosome inside the cells (girls are XX, boys are XY).

But tests that require the removal of cells carry slight risks of causing an abortion, so they are almost never used simply to determine sex. And, even though you can know your little bundle of joy's gender even before the stork has dropped the bundle, there is nothing you can do, short of ending the pregnancy, if you're not happy.

That is about to change. There are now 57 clinics in the United States, along with eight in other countries, that are offering a technique allowing would-be parents to pick their baby's gender. A Montana-based company, Gametrics Limited, has patented a process that uses artificial insemination to increase the odds of having a boy or a girl.

The key to the technique involves having sperm swim through a test tube filled with a specially prepared gel. The sperm that make it to the bottom are more likely to have a Y (male) chromosome. So, depending on what the parents want, the woman is artificially inseminated with sperm from the top or the bottom of the test tube.

The technique is not new. The founder of Gametrics, Ronald J. Ericsson, first reported on his sperm separation technique in 1973. But others have had a hard time replicating Ericsson's results.

Ericsson and two colleagues, Ferdinand Beernink of the East Baby Fertility Group in Berkeley, Calif., and W. Paul Dmowski of Chicago's Rush Medical College, say they can prove the technique has worked well in a large number of births at a variety of clinics.

At the 65 Sperm Centers franchised to offer Ericsson's technique, couples beat the roughly 50-50 odds associated with making babies the old-fashioned way. Those who wanted a boy were successful in 749 out of 1,034 births. That is a 72 percent success rate. Ericsson and his group reported similar success rates for those seeking girls: 133 out of 193 pregnancies produced girls, a success rate of 69 percent.

There are lots of reasons why people might want to select their babies' sex. Some of them make a great deal of moral sense. Certain diseases, such as hemophilia, are linked to sex. Couples who know they are at risk of having a child with a sex-linked genetic disease could prevent a good deal of suffering and premature death by picking their baby's gender.

The technique might also help some couples who now have more children than they really want in the hope that the next one will be a different sex from those they already have.

But other reasons for sex selection are not morally commendable. In many societies, such as China and India, there are strong cultural biases against females. The bias is so strong that some experts believe thousands of female babies are killed each year in China.

In the United States preferences for boys over girls do not appear to be as strong. Various surveys of married men and women over the past 20 years show that there is a small preference for boys over girls for the first child. However, that when a couple already has a boy, there is a very strong preference that the next child be a girl.

Americans have spent a great deal of time arguing about whether women ought to be permitted to serve in combat or work as firefighters and in other occupations.

Medical science is about to put our talk of equal opportunity and gender equality to a much more severe test. If we can live up to our rhetoric and really value men and women equally, then sex selection will only enhance the joy of having a baby. But if gender prejudice is still deeply rooted in society, then removing the mystery about the sex of our offspring will be no cause for joy.

Brave New Babies

Few topics fascinate us as much as the emerging techniques for making babies. And why shouldn't they? Reproductive technology has it all—sex, science and the potential for sin.

Manipulating sperm, eggs and embryos takes us about as close as we can get to controlling our destiny. But the current crop of reproductive techniques—artificial insemination, *in vitro* fertilization, embryo transfer, frozen embryos, gamete interfallopian transfer, embryo biopsy—leaves us capable of little more than scratching our collective moral head as we decide how those advances should be used, who should have access to them and how we should readjust our notions of parenthood and family.

But just wait; you ain't seen nothin' yet. You don't believe me? Then come along on a trip into the not-so-distant future for a taste of the moral and legal challenges that await your grandchildren. The following may seem like science fiction; but it's extrapolated from research that is actually going on right now.

The year is 2040. You are a 14-year-old girl. You've just used the home gene-probe kit that you got in your sex-education class for your weekly screen. It shows you are pregnant and that the embryo is a girl.

Now, you can't understand how this happened. Your boyfriend is taking a pill that is supposed to keep him from making sperm. And you have a tiny implant in your arm that is supposed to make it impossible for ovulation to occur.

But the test can't be wrong. You are the one in 600,000 cases where the contraceptives fail. What on earth are you going to tell your parents?

You're afraid that your father will be furious and will make you sue the implant manufacturer. Your mother will never believe that your boyfriend was taking his pills. And your parents are sure to give you the standard speech about how an unlicensed pregnancy can jeopardize your chances at getting student loans, early-retirement benefits or government jobs.

If you want to continue the pregnancy, you will need to go with one or your parents to get a waiver from a judge. You know that the pressure to end your pregnancy will be enormous.

Even so, you finally break down and tell Mom. She schedules your appointment with the genitrician. The doctor threads a full-color, three-dimensional ultrasound stethoscope into your uterus and examines the tiny embryo growing there.

While everything looks OK, she follows standard procedure and collects a few cells from the fetus's foot and the amniotic fluid. She inserts these into her office GENALYZER, which automatically isolates the chromosomes, splits them and matches the component DNA against a standard map of the human genome.

Your embryo scores nine out of a possible 10 on the Watson-Hood-Chugai Genetic Risk Scale. The female fetus's genetic risks are slightly higher than average for diabetes if she doesn't watch her weight after menopause, and there's a disposition toward alcoholism, which is easily correctable by supplementing her post-birth diet with a metabolism enhancer for a few years.

There is no medical basis for terminating this pregnancy. Still, you're going to have to decide what you want to do with your embryo. And you're going to have to decide quickly. The four-week viability period is almost over.

Your mother says that you absolutely must have the fetus flushed at the nearby Fetal Care Unit at Sinai/Lutheran. But you insist that the decision is yours to make—and you have the law on your side.

You know that your boyfriend will go along with whatever you decide. He assigns custody to you or to whichever agency arranges the embryo adoption.

Having a baby would be nice, but you're afraid of what a pregnancy entails—dietary supplements, the hyper-oxygen pills, the metabolic balancers, the nuisance of the implantable fetal monitor and stimulator, the chore of swallowing anti-virals every day. Natural pregnancy is no picnic. And that's why the government subsidizes the fetal care units.

In the end, you opt for the flush. Mom schedules the appointment for you and gets the credits shifted from the government fund to the family fund to cover the costs. The embryo will be painlessly flushed from your womb directly into an extra-corporeal artificial uterus, where it will be brought to term under the watchful eyes of the well-trained team of fetologists.

These dedicated doctors and nurses will take care of inserting the artificial microislet cells that will compensate for the embryo's propensity to diabetes. They also will arrange placement with a family or individual looking to adopt through one of the various parental benevolent associations. You'll be able to leave the clinic knowing that quick placement for a "niner," like this embryo, will not be a problem.

Had enough of the trip to tomorrowland? If you think the current crop of reproductive technologies is remarkable or raises tough moral questions, stay tuned for the next 50 years.

In 1990, the available techniques for intervening in reproduction are still incredibly primitive. For example, some drugs can be used to help people create viable eggs and sperm—but when these do not work, we turn to substituting someone else's egg or sperm. In the future, the only reason to use someone else's reproductive materials will be if someone is absolutely sterile or has a major hereditary disease that is beyond repair.

Current reproductive technologies consist of the manipulation of embryos during the first few days of life. After that, development cannot be sustained. But the field of neonatology has made incredible advances in lowering the age of viability for fetuses. It is not unusual to hear of babies alive today who were born at only 23 or 24 weeks gestational age.

At some point in the next century, neonatology will intersect with the field of fertility treatment. We will have the ability to bring embryos to term outside a woman's body. When that day comes, the notion of natural childbirth will be quickly replaced with the question of whether natural pregnancy is preferable to artificial pregnancy.

To date, advances in genetics have barely touched reproductive technology. But as the capacity to keep an embryo alive outside the womb evolves, the prospects for screening and altering the hereditary makeup of that embryo will evolve as well. The central moral question of the 21st century will be the degree to which genetic risk should influence decisions about bringing embryos to term.

No story appears on television or in the newspaper today about *in vitro* fertilization, surrogate motherhood or embryo transfer without the obligatory hand-wringing as to how medicine is moving so fast that ethics and law cannot keep pace. And in one sense, this is true. Our society has reached no political, legal or moral consensus about what to do about the wonders of the current generation of reproductive technologies.

Our courts are clogged with all sorts of nasty spats as to who gets custody of the baby that resulted when eggs were obtained from Mrs. A who gave them to Ms. B who fertilized them with sperm from her ex-husband, Mr. C, who gave the resulting embryo to Miss D who, hired under the auspices of a contract issued by Mr. E, head of a small surrogate-mother firm, carried the embryo to term for Mr. and Mrs. F.

But the inability to reach consensus about these conundrums does not mean that it is impossible to foresee where the ethical issues will lie as reproductive technology continues to advance. Ethics is not so intellectually flabby that it cannot keep pace with medicine by pinpointing the ethical dilemmas of tomorrow.

The problem is that the future of baby-making is so startling, so unfamiliar, so just plain spooky that our society finds it hard to look directly at what technology promises to make possible. We are so comfortable with our outdated economic, legal, social, familial and cultural institutions and arrangements that we are afraid to ask whether they will be capable of absorbing 21st century modes of making babies.

CHAPTER 3
RELATIONSHIPS BETWEEN HEALTH CARE
PROVIDERS AND THOSE IN THEIR CARE

Jargon Used in Hospitals Reveals
Ambivalence Care-Givers Feel

I am not a big fan of the word police. You know, William Safire, James J. Kilpatrick, Ed Neumann and their ilk—men and women with bodies artificially pumped up beyond recognition by years of thesaurus lifting.

These are folks with a serious case of priorities out of whack. The desire of verbal fussbudgets to impose a "new word order" upon an American language brimming with argot, jargon and, best of all, slang, leaves me ice cold. Language should be examined, not to prune and trim it like a bonsai tree, but to revel in its richness and diversity.

Language prudes fail to appreciate the varied delights of the verbal stew that is constantly bubbling up all around us. The most intolerant members of this cult also fail to understand that argot and jargon are rich in clues and insights into what people really value and what issues disturb and trouble them.

Nowhere is this more evident than in the slang and jargon that permeate daily professional conversations in hospitals and nursing homes.

When today's young doctors and nurses care for patients whom they do not like, especially those who are sick as a result of abusing drugs or booze, they grumble that a "gomer" (get out of my emergency room) or "dirtball" has fallen into their laps.

Patients who come into hospital emergency rooms with multiple injuries and medical problems are "trainwrecks."

Little kids in the intensive care nursery who do not seem to be doing well for no obvious reason are suffering from FTT—"failure to thrive."

When a young resident or fellow is not sure exactly what is wrong with a new patient, they pay a "kick the tires visit."

"Spiking a fever" is a possible sign of infection. And where cancer is involved, "mets" to the brain or liver (metastases, or the spread of cancer cells) is very bad news.

When patients are critically ill, everyone monitors test results carefully to see whether or not an infection is going to "tip the patient over"—whether they will survive or not.

The most revealing language can be found in the intensive care unit. An elderly patient who is admitted with "chartomegaly," a large stack of thick medical records from previous hospitalizations, has a very poor chance of surviving a stay in intensive care.

Subjecting a patient to high-tech aggressive care such as ventilators, numerous diagnostic tests, artificial feeding and kidney dialysis is commonly and tellingly referred to as "flogging the patient." Someone receiving maximal care in intensive care is sometimes referred to as a "technopatient."

If a patient isn't hacking it despite all the best efforts of the intensive care staff, the patient is "circling the drain." When that happens, it is not unusual for lots of superspecialists, or "buzzards," to appear at the bedside.

If the buzzards can't figure out what is wrong and death is inevitable, then it is time to "dial down" the ventilator in order to allow the patient to die. This may require "snowing" the patient—giving high doses of morphine—to relieve pain.

Most patients die "euboxic," with all their biochemical measures normal (all boxes for minimal physical functions on their chart checked off), even though their heart, brain or lungs give out, since our health care system has a very hard time letting patients die.

The language cops would certainly be appalled to see what doctors and nurses do to the language in the privacy of the workplace. But while the grammar may be flawed and the terminology opaque to the outsider, the medical slang tossed around in the hospital trenches shows just how uneasy doctors and nurses feel about the value of what they do in our emergency rooms and intensive care units and their doubts about what it does to the patients who receive it.

It may offend some ears to hear that dirtballs and technopatients are common terms among healers who work in these settings. But the language reveals the values crisis that simmers just beneath the surface in these places as health care professionals vent their anger and ambivalence.

No one wants to think of Mom or Dad as being flogged by medical technology, but the reality is that there does come a time as the doctors and nurses know when "aggressive care" becomes more aggressive than caring.

If you want to understand what is wrong with our health care system, don't limit yourself to the good grammar on display in medical publications.

Listen carefully to the way doctors and nurses actually talk to one another about their patients and their work. The jargon of our healers tells us a lot about the moral and emotional ambivalence that is at epidemic levels in such places.

In Health Care Reform Think of
Patient Comfort Too

My father-in-law, Robert Stojak, died of colon cancer. He spent his final weeks in a hospital bed, which afforded me an unwanted but important perspective on how well the health care system deals with terminally ill patients.

First the good news—a good deal of progress has been made in allowing terminally ill patients to control the use of medical technology. Doctors were generally very willing to abide by my father-in-law's wishes about aggressive medical care. He said he did not want any extraordinary forms of life-support or heroic measures and none were given. It was not hard to get agreement on a "no resuscitation" order once that time had come.

Those who think that there are large sums of money to be saved by encouraging the more conservative use of high technology on dying patients may not realize that clinical practice is already moving rapidly in this direction.

Now the bad news. It was not the life and death decisions but, the routine, mundane activities of hospital care that were a source of ethical vexation. None of his doctors really wanted to tell him that he was terminally ill.

I finally asked him what he wanted to know and, when he said everything, we spent a couple of hours talking about his diagnosis and what he could expect in the time that remained.

Once he got over his shock and sorrow, he went so far as to tell me about his will and what he wanted in the way of a funeral, since he was very concerned that his death not be a burden to his wife and family.

Those in white coats are not the only folks who have a hard time addressing the subject of death. When the topic of hospice or home care arose, I told my mother-in-law to call her church to find out how to make arrangements.

Despite the fact the hospice was church-affiliated, local church officials did not have a clue about what to do. I asked other clergy who came to visit about hospice and they too were at a loss. There is absolutely no excuse for leaving talk of hospice and home care for the dying to doctors.

The doctors and nurses were, on the whole, good people who did an outstanding job of caring for their patients. But our hospitals are ridden with microethical problems that grate incessantly on a patient and family's nerves.

The delivery of three meals a day for weeks to a man who could not possibly eat a morsel would have been funny if it were not so sad. Chairs that would support a visitor comfortably for an hour when they needed to be occupied eight or 10 hours a day drove me nuts. Promises to be back in a minute to do something that were followed by mysterious, unexplained disappearances that stretched into hours left many a family member seething.

The major source of these little irritants is that doctors and nurses are too busy. The pace they follow creates an environment that is as caustic to human feelings as cancer is to the human body. It sometimes took a busy nurse more than half an hour to administer a shot to relieve pain.

Senior physicians spend less than a minute in a patient's room when they visit and they are too harried to visit very often. A family member with a question stands a much better chance of finding the doctor by hanging out near an elevator instead of the patient's room.

A good rule to follow about hospitals is never, ever go alone. If you are very ill, someone needs to be present to act as your advocate, gofer and confidant. A good corollary to follow is don't go on a weekend. Staffing drops to a minimum and students are in charge.

The work level of big hospitals creates a huge problem for the coordination of information about each patient's diagnosis and treatment plans. Nurses coming on a new shift, or, who are part-timers working on a weekend, often have no idea of the patient's status or what the doctor is planning to do next.

The doctors themselves are not always on the same page. It is easy to see why, since beepers, pagers and answering services are always beckoning. When calls are not returned for seven or eight hours, then work load levels have risen well beyond what patients have a right to expect.

One of the nastiest problems in hospitals is the continuing parade of persons who have tasks to do in the patient's room. Garbage is taken out, mail delivered, newspapers hawked, cable TV adjusted, food brought in, vital signs measured, baths administered—the parade of humanity is uncoordinated and neverending. My brother-in-law and I counted 24 entries in one eight-hour weekday shift.

Add to this stream of humankind the fact that lights and noise in a room with two sick people in it rarely dim and you have created a perfect sleep-free zone.

Backbreaking work loads in combination with cold, institutional environments can go a long way toward defeating the best of intentions and the most indomitable of spirits. As we begin the task of reforming our health care system, we owe it to patients to try to make one that is not only more cost-effective but a lot more user-friendly.

Should We Lie to Mom
About Alzheimer's?

Imagine that you suspect that your mother has Alzheimer's disease. For many months, you have noticed her having trouble understanding conversations. Activities that used to bring her pleasure are rapidly becoming sources of frustration and anger. She is having serious problems remembering certain things.

You decide that you had better take her to a doctor. But you are afraid of what might happen if the diagnosis is Alzheimer's. Your mom always has been a very proud and independent person. She would not take kindly to the news that she is going to slowly lose her mind.

The thought crosses your mind that she might even try to kill herself. You decide that you had better call the doctor first to make sure that if the news is bad, you will be told but your mother will not.

Should the doctor honor your request? That's the tough question addressed in a provocative article in the April 2, 1992 issue of the *New England Journal of Medicine*. Margaret Drickamer and Mark Lachs, physicians who treat Alzheimer's patients and their families at the West Haven (Conn.) Veterans Hospital and the Yale-New Haven Hospital, suggest that sometimes it is right to withhold from the patient a diagnosis of Alzheimer's.

The doctors' arguments for keeping an Alzheimer's diagnosis secret from a patient fall into three major categories: uncertainty, harm and incompetency. I think only the last is a valid reason.

The clinical diagnosis of Alzheimer's disease cannot be made with *absolute* certainty without a post-mortem autopsy. Even when a patient has serious and obvious symptoms, the diagnosis is wrong about 10 percent of the time. The diagnosis is even harder to make in the earliest stages of the disease. Even when the diagnosis is correct, the rate of mental deterioration varies from patient to patient.

Uncertainty is a fact of life with Alzheimer's; it is not a reason for the doctor to withhold the truth. Not being sure is not going to stop your mother or mine from drawing her own diagnostic conclusions, despite what the doctor does or doesn't say. As doctors who treat patients with cancer have long known, patients are very good at guessing what the doctor is afraid to say.

OK, but shouldn't the doctor consider that the diagnosis of Alzheimer's may depress someone like your mother—even lead to her suicide? Even if these risks are real, are they really arguments against telling the truth or, rather, about the need for care and caution in doing so? The truth can hurt. Those who deal with Alzheimer's, as well as those who pay for their health care, must do a better job of making the time and resources available to teach those who diagnose or have Alzheimer's how to cope with the truth.

People with Alzheimer's are often going to be, as Drickamer and Lachs note, depressed, agitated, paranoid and upset. But lying itself will put an emotional burden on the patient, who will not understand why his or her family is so upset.

Alzheimer's does provide one reason for the doctor to be less than honest: Those who have the disease may have lost the ability to understand the diagnosis. I cannot see how it would be anything but cruel to try to convey a diagnosis to a person who is seriously demented.

Family members often think they can cope better than the person who's sick when the news from the doctor is grim. However, competent people, especially your own mother, deserve the right, if they choose to exercise it, to grapple with their infirmities.

Alzheimer's may steal the mind, but it should not be permitted to kill the truth for those who want to know it.

Hospital Can "Give the Boot" to Drug Abuser

A man—I'll call him Paul Smith—was discharged last week from a hospital in California. But "discharge" is a polite term to describe the circumstances of his departure. "Booted out the door" gets a lot closer to the truth.

Smith's doctors and nurses to not believe that the street is the best place for him to be. Yet, they agreed he ought to leave the hospital. In fact, they insisted on it.

Smith was in the hospital because he had been stabbed in a fight with another man over drugs. While there, he received a visit from an old pal from his neighborhood. A few hours later, a nurse found Smith mumbling and nodding off in his room. She guessed he was high.

The nurse called a physician, and they asked Smith if he had used narcotics. Initially, he simply refused to talk. But under persistent questioning, he admitted that his visitor was a heroin dealer who had not dropped by to inquire about his health.

When Smith's next routine blood test was done, the doctor ordered a test for drugs—without telling him. The test came back positive for heroin. The physician went right back to Smith and told him that hospital security was going to come into the room and search for drugs. If the search turned up any, he would get one more chance to stay clean. But if he abused drugs again, he would be discharged.

Hospital security searched Smith's room. He told them to leave, but they ignored him. They found a small bag of heroin in the back of a drawer in his bedside table. They took it and left.

During the next few days, a few other "friends" stopped by Smith's room. None of the hospital staff saw anything suspicious in these visits, but drug screens continued to be run, still unbeknownst to Smith. Eight days later, his blood tested positive for both heroin and PCP (angel dust).

At that point, a nurse came in and told Smith that he was being discharged. He protested, saying he was too sick to leave and that he was not using drugs. His doctor told him he was lying; his blood tests showed that he was using.

Smith received a quick lesson in how to administer antibiotics through his IV line. He was told that a social worker would visit his house in a day or two to see how he was doing.

Then, security personnel came back to the room, packed up his possessions, wheeled him to the front door, yanked him out of the wheelchair and left him yelling and swearing in the street.

Should the medical staff have tossed out Paul Smith?

One of the worst breaches of ethics a doctor or nurse can commit is patient abandonment. Still, how much nonsense must doctors and nurses endure? Patients have responsibilities as well as rights.

I do not approve of the way in which Smith's blood was surreptitiously tested or the way his room was searched, but I do think the hospital staff was right to discharge him. Doctors and nurses must not discharge patients if they know those patients will die outside the hospital. But that is not true in this case. Smith was sent packing when he broke the terms for receiving hospital care. The staff made arrangements to see him at home, which while not as desirable as keeping him in the hospital was nonetheless not abandoning him.

Hospitals are not prisons, but neither are they shooting galleries. In order to enjoy rights, patients must agree not to continue to hurt themselves and to abide by the rules of the hospital. If they don't, their right to be there ends.

Trainers, Doctors Owe Athletes
Guidance on Blood Doping

The *Journal of Laboratory and Clinical Medicine* is not the sort of publication you would expect to find in a high school locker room or the lounge of an athletic dormitory on a college campus.

That's too bad, because the September, 1992 issue contains two articles that present information that might mean the difference between life and death. The articles also raise some tough ethical questions for physicians, trainers and coaches who work with athletes.

The subject under discussion in the *Journal* is blood doping. Blood doping—or, as it is sometimes called, "liquid aerobics"—refers to any activity that can boost the ability of the blood to carry oxygen.

The trick to increased oxygen capacity—and thus, increased endurance—is to get more red cells into the blood. This can be done by training at high altitude, which makes the body produce more red cells, getting transfusions of red cells (your own or somebody else's) or by taking a new drug, recombinant human erythropoietin, which allows the body to make lots more red cells.

Two Canadian researchers, Delia Roberts and D.J. Smith, who are at the Human Performance Laboratory at the University of Calgary, report the results of their examination of the effects of just three weeks of training at high altitude on nine world-class Canadian swimmers.

The Canadian researchers found that a sudden switch to altitude training carries a price. All of the swimmers in the study experienced significant losses in the iron levels of their blood, some as much as 50 percent.

Low levels of iron in the body can have serious health consequences. Competitive athletes, especially young ones, often can see only the benefits and are not interested in hearing about risks, where getting an advantage through modifying training techniques is concerned.

Doctors, trainers and athletic officials have a duty to make sure that the risks are both heard and minimized.

Not all doctors, trainers and coaches are as morally scrupulous as they ought to be when it comes to protecting the health of athletes. That is clear from the other article in the journal, a disturbing review of artificial blood doping written by a physician, E. Randy Eichner from the University of Oklahoma Health Sciences Center.

Does blood doping work? Dr. Eichner thinks so. Study after study has shown that anything that can build up the number of red cells in the blood—whether it is training at altitude, transfusions or using drugs to stimulate red cell production—provides a slight improvement in performance.

Slight improvements may only amount to a second or two, but that can be the difference between winning and losing.

Do athletes know about blood doping? As Dr. Eichner notes, "When science marches on, elite athletes—always seeking an edge—are never far behind."

Pre-race transfusions may seem an especially unappetizing way to eke out a victory. This has led to the latest and scariest development in blood doping. According to Dr. Eichner, the latest trend in blood doping is drugs.

From 1987 to 1990, 18 Belgian and Dutch cyclists, athletes in prime condition, dropped dead suddenly and unexpectedly. Rumors abound that these athletes were fooling around with recombinant human erythropoietin (rhEPO).

In other words, they were using drugs to boost their red cell volumes in order to get a competitive endurance advantage in their long and arduous races.

Eichner thinks that rhEPO carries enormous risks. Not only will the drug make red blood cells; it also can raise your blood pressure and increase the viscosity of your blood to the point where a stroke or a fatal thrombosis in the lung becomes a very real danger.

Do bicyclists and other competitive athletes want to hear about these risks? Hardly. The saying on the European cycling tour when the subject turns to matters such as using drugs to blood dope is "Better dead than second."

Blood doping puts the ethics of doctors, trainers and coaches to the test precisely because it works. Athletes may well say they understand the risks associated with the practice of blood doping or other pharmacological means of improving performance such as steroids or growth hormone. It is tempting to say that all the doctor or trainer need do is present the risk and then let the chips fall where they may.

Such an attitude is understandable, but it is not ethical. A doctor, coach or trainer has no obligation to allow athletes to take risks that will cause long-term harm or death, especially young athletes whose view of risk is colored by their own perception that they are immortal. It is the job of the doctor, coach and trainer to balance the desire to win against the costs involved.

When the subject is blood doping, paternalism is no vice.

Doctors Should Study Killers,
Not Help with Executions

Just before Christmas, 1992, the American Medical Association declared participation by physicians in executions unethical.

Thirty-seven states have the death penalty. The demand for doctors to monitor vital signs, provide lethal injections or drugs, supervise others involved in administering the death penalty or declaring death has been increasing as more and more prisoners are executed.

I think the AMA did the right thing. But no case puts that view to the test more than the repulsive criminal career of Westley Allan Dodd. If there was ever a need for a poster boy for the death penalty Westley Allan Dodd would do just fine.

In 1989 Dodd, then 28-years-old, confessed to authorities in the state of Washington that he had stabbed to death two brothers, Cole and William Neer. He also admitted repeatedly raping and then killing Lee Iseli. Lee Iseli was four. The Cole brothers were ten and eleven when Dodd killed them.

Consistently violent career criminals are hard to find. Dodd is one. His rampage of rape and abuse began when he was thirteen. He sexually molested two of his cousins. Throughout high school he was arrested several times for molesting children.

In 1981 he was discharged from the Navy when the cops caught him offering money to boys for sex. Further arrests for sex offenses against minors followed in the states of Idaho and Washington. Dodd has seen many therapists over the years both in and out of jail. He says he was never serious about treatment for his molesting.

He told Washington state court officials that "Each time I entered treatment, I continued to molest children. I liked molesting children and did what I had to do to avoid jail so I could continue molesting."

Dodd is without remorse. He laughs at doctors, social workers and psychologists who seek to help him. Last year he told a Washington state court that the state had to kill him.

In waiving any appeal of his death sentence he wrote, "I must be executed before I have an opportunity to escape and kill someone else. If I do escape I promise you I will kill and rape again and I will enjoy every minute of it."

Considering the misery he has left in his wake, it is hard to resist the urge to want Dodd dead. The declarations of doctors that they will not participate in executions seems frivolous in the face of what a man like Dodd has done to children.

But the AMA position is right. Dodd says that the state had better execute him or else. Why should we permit someone like Dodd to threaten us from his jail cell? Where does a man like this come off claiming the right to drag others down to his level of moral bestiality by demanding that they must hang him, gas him or give him a lethal injection?

Dodd has spent most of his life coercing children. Is the right punishment to permit him and others like him to coerce the medical, legal and prison authorities to wallow in his trough of violence and death?

Criminals like Dodd need to be studied, not killed. We need to understand what makes them tick so that we can stop them before they molest, rape and kill. And, criminals like a Westley Allan Dodd should not be permitted to threaten or bully the medical community or anyone else into doing their bidding.

Dodd wants to die. Should we do him the honor of fulfilling his request? Or is a more fitting punishment forcing him to live in a maximum security prison in isolation while experts try to learn why he is what he is?

When doctors refuse to participate in executions they do so because they do not believe that their skills should be used to achieve the aims of the criminal justice system. They are right. Doctors should not kill on the orders of the state. Nor should the state allow incorrigible, violent criminals to have any say in their punishment.

What would serve society best is to understand the Westley Allan Dodds of this world in order to prevent them. What would punish such criminals is knowing that biomedical science intends to use them for society's interest rather than allowing them to use medicine for theirs.

Donor Decision Made in the Heart
Not in the Courts

Jean-Pierre Bosze is 12 years old. He is dying of leukemia. His only hope of survival is a bone-marrow transplant.

In the fall of 1992, Monica Reynolds, a judge in Chicago, told the boy and his father, Tamas, that she would not force the two people who are in the best position to help Jean-Pierre to be tested to determine if they actually could.

She made the right decision. The potential bone-marrow donors for Jean-Pierre are his twin half-sister and half-brother. They are 3-1/2 years old.

The twins live with their mother, Nancy Curran. Tamas Bosze had a relationship with Curran during a time when he was estranged from his wife, Jean-Pierre's mother. That relationship resulted in the birth of the twins.

Because bone-marrow transplants work best when performed using biologically related donors, the twins are the most likely candidates to help Jean-Pierre—although the odds are still less than one in a thousand that either is an exact match. Bosze and his wife already have been tested, but they do not match their son's marrow type.

Curran has refused to have the twins tested to see if they are compatible donors for Jean-Pierre. It is not clear why. Perhaps she is refusing because her relationship with Bosze went sour and he is back with his wife. She could be furious because Bosze apparently initially denied paternity of the twins. Or she may simply not want the twins—either of them—to serve as a donor because she does not want to put them through the marrow-procurement procedure.

Marrow donation is not especially dangerous, but it does involve more rigmarole than blood donation. The donor must stay overnight in a hospital. General anesthesia is used when marrow is taken from the hip. The donor experiences some soreness in the hips and back for a few days, on the order of that produced by a bad bruise. And transfusions may be needed if too much blood is lost when the marrow is removed.

No one has ever died donating marrow, but general anesthesia does carry a tiny risk of death, as do blood transfusions in the age of AIDS and hepatitis.

Whether a court should force the twins to be tested in the face of their mother's refusal to consent has few legal precedents. However, in 1978, a Pennsylvania judge refused to order a Pittsburgh man, David Shimp, to donate marrow to his cousin, Robert McFall, who was dying of aplastic anemia. McFall had undergone radiation therapy to destroy his own marrow on the basis of his cousin's promise that he would donate. But Shimp had second thoughts and backed out of the procedure.

Unless the court forced a donation, McFall could die immediately, since he had no marrow at all. The court called the suddenly reluctant Shimp a lot of names but, in the end, refused to force him to undergo surgery solely for the benefit of another person. McFall died a few days later.

The same principle that guided the Pennsylvania court applies in the Bosze case. Courts should not force anyone to undergo medical tests or procedures intended only to benefit another individual. It is certainly right to help someone in need, but there is no legal basis to force someone to do what is right—especially when that someone is 3-1/2 years old.

Tamas Bosze appealed Judge Reynolds' decision not to compel testing. But it is hard to imagine any court in America ordering nontherapeutic medical tests on minor children over the objection of their mother—whatever her reasons may be.

There is another way to find a potential marrow donor for this young boy. Jean-Pierre's best hope lies not in a courtroom but in the altruism of strangers. If each of us is willing to sign up as a prospective donor with the National Marrow Donor Program, based in St. Paul, Jean Pierre may yet find a donor. It is very hard to find marrow donors among strangers, but the odds of finding a match increase as more volunteers agree to serve.

Ironically, Nancy Curran's choice concerning testing is not confined to her twins. She must decide if she is willing to be tested since—although the odds are very long—she might turn out to be a compatible donor. The ultimate solution to the dilemma of children such as Jean-Pierre hinges on whether each one of us is willing to volunteer to do what a court—quite correctly—is not willing to force a 3-1/2-year-old to do.

It May be Waste, But It's Still Ours to Control

Every year, millions of women give birth in hospitals all over the United States. When a full-term birth occurs, more than a baby arrives. A placenta, an umbilical cord and a variety of fluids are delivered as well.

Few of us spend any time pondering the fate of the tissues that constitute the uterine support system. Most of us have no desire to look at all that stuff, much less worry about what happens to it. But as the biotechnology revolution marches ahead, that attitude may change.

Scientists have realized that the umbilical cord is a good source of endothelial cells. These cells act as a barrier or filter between blood and other tissues. As such, they are of special interest to researchers, since they can be used to mimic processes that take place in the bloodstream and as models for studying the effects of various drugs. Scientists interested in studying endothelial cells get them by scraping the lining of the umbilical cord and then growing the cells artificially.

The system that has evolved for obtaining umbilical cords is very simple. Researchers call hospitals where there are large numbers of births and ask the obstetrical nurses to save some of the umbilical cords for them rather than sending them off to the incinerator. Once in a while, the researchers drop off some coffee and doughnuts to thank the nurses for their efforts.

But in some parts of the country, coffee and doughnuts no longer suffice. Some private, commercial medical companies—among them, Bio-Vascular, a firm based in Minnesota—have found new uses for umbilical cords. Bio-Vascular has developed methods for modifying human umbilical cords so that the veins they contain can be used in bypass operations, especially for people who have circulatory problems in their legs. In 1989, Bio-Vascular sold $1.5 million worth of modified human umbilical cords.

Officials at Bio-Vascular were not willing to talk with me about their system for obtaining cords. But informed sources tell me that the company obtains a large number of umbilical cords by paying $5 to $10 per cord.

There are at least two other companies that are paying hospitals to provide them with umbilical cords.

During a telephone interview, Carl Southerland, director of research at Cell Systems in Kirkland, Wash., said his company has been using cords to grow endothelial cell lines since the early 1970s. The cell lines are sold to researchers. The hospitals where the cords are obtained have recently introduced consent forms asking parents to sign away any claim of ownership to these "waste" materials.

Umbilical cords are not the only tissues being transformed from waste to valuable commodities. Cells from placentas and foreskins removed during circumcisions also are used to create cell lines that are sometimes sold for large profits. And in several hospitals in the United States, prospective parents are asked to sell blood from the umbilical cord. The blood contains substances that have many potential uses, including transplantation for those needing bone-marrow cells.

Is the evolution of a market in human waste unethical? Is it wrong for companies to pay hospitals for tissues that would otherwise be destroyed? And how is anyone harmed when companies manufacture medically valuable substances from material that otherwise has no value to the person from whose body it came?

If the market for placentas, umbilical cords, fluids and other biological materials continues to expand—and there is every reason to think it will—we need to establish the right to control the fate of our biological wastes.

The fact that scientists now can transform biological waste into substances of value merits applause, not condemnation. But those who want these materials are under an obligation to get explicit permission for their use. And this entails giving parents a full range of options.

So many babies are born each year that no one is likely to make a big profit from selling an umbilical cord or a foreskin. But if we want to demand payment for such things, we should have the right to do that. If we would rather donate them freely to medical research or to commercial companies, we should have that right to do that. Or if we want them to be destroyed or disposed of in some other way, that is our right as well.

The social good that can come from the biological wizardry that allows junk to be transformed into treasure must be balanced against the desire some people may have to determine the fate of their own and their children's tissues.

CHAPTER 4
THE RIGHT TO REFUSE MEDICAL TREATMENT

Anencephaly Case: No Cure,
Just Prolonging of Death

Can a hospital turn off a baby's life-saving medical technology against the wishes of the child's mother? A federal judge in Virginia in the case of an infant known only as Baby K says "no." That may not be a wise decision.

The events leading to the court ruling began when Baby K's mother—referred to in the court's decision as Ms. H—was told a few months into her pregnancy that her baby had a condition known as anencephaly. This is a birth defect in which most of the brain does not develop.

A child with anencephaly cannot think, feel anything, see, talk or hear. Too much of the brain is missing to allow the child to ever be conscious.

An obstetrician and neonatologist advised Ms. H to terminate the pregnancy. She refused. Baby K was born via cesarean section on Oct. 13, 1992. Baby K did have anencephaly. The baby also had trouble breathing. So the physicians temporarily put her on a mechanical ventilator. They wanted the mom to have a chance to say good-bye to the baby.

Within a few days, the doctors asked Ms. H to allow them not to use the ventilator the next time Baby K had trouble breathing. They said Baby K's condition was absolutely hopeless. They had no treatment or cure. It was only a matter of time before she would die.

The mother would not give the approval the doctors sought to let her baby die. She insisted her baby be put on a ventilator whenever she appeared to have difficulty breathing. She said that she firmly believed that all human life has value, that life must be protected and that God might work a miracle with her baby.

The doctors were astonished. They did not believe that they were accomplishing anything by keeping a child with anencephaly on life-support. They told the mother again and again that putting Baby K on a ventilator was pointless, futile and completely inappropriate. The hospital's ethics committee agreed. But the mother still insisted on care.

The hospital administration then decided that the next time Baby K was stable enough to come off the respirator, they would transfer her to another facility.

On Nov. 30, 1992, she was moved to a nearby nursing home. But Baby K was brought back to the hospital twice in the next four months when she suffered severe breathing problems.

On March 15, the doctors—convinced they would never get the mother's permission to stop the use of the ventilator—did a tracheotomy in which they surgically implanted a tube into Baby K's windpipe to make it easier to put her on and off the breathing machine. They also asked a court to appoint a guardian for Baby K.

The guardian and the child's father both agreed that the next time she had severe trouble breathing, Baby K ought to be allowed to die. But Ms. H did not. So the baby went back to the nursing home.

Baby K is still in the nursing home and Ms. H is still insisting that the ventilator be used whenever it looks like her breathing might stop. The hospital has now been told by the Virginia court that it must follow the mother's wishes.

The court reached this opinion by noting that under a newly enacted federal law, the Emergency Medical Treatment and Active Labor Act, it is illegal for a hospital not to treat someone brought to a hospital in an emergency medical condition.

Since the law makes no exceptions and another federal law, the Rehabilitation Act of 1973, explicitly prohibits discrimination on the basis of handicap, then the hospital would be breaking the law if it did not put Baby K on a respirator. An inability to breathe is a medical emergency and Baby K is handicapped, the court held.

The problem with the court's reasoning is that it stretches definitions to classify anencephaly as a disability. Yes, it is true that a child born with most of its brain missing is severely limited in what it can do. But a child with most of its brain missing is not disabled; it is unabled.

A human being who has permanently lost all capacity to think, feel, sense, interact or be in any way aware of their surroundings or who was born without all of these abilities is someone beyond the help of medical science.

No parent wants to hear that medicine has nothing to offer a child dying of a terrible disorder. But surely our legislators cannot really have intended to mandate that children with anencephaly must be kept alive regardless of the resources required, regardless of the fact that the treatment does absolutely nothing to alter the severity of the condition, regardless of the fact that it is impossible for the child to even know that treatment is being given or that a mother cares.

Parents, as the court notes in its decision, ought to have the right to decide the care of their child. But medicine must be allowed to say what is beyond the realm of medical possibility.

God may yet work a miracle in the case of Baby K. But if that happens, a mechanical ventilator will not be needed. Doctors need to use technology like ventilators to maintain life. Society needs to grant doctors some discretion about when the use of technology is simply prolonging death.

Laws Shouldn't Interfere with Keri Lynn's Life

I got a call from Dave Andrusko, the editor of *National Right to Life News* and, at times, an intellectual sparring partner of mine on bioethical issues. He told me about a newspaper story about a little girl who once was at the heart of a landmark bioethics controversy—Baby Jane Doe.

Andrusko believed time had proven him right and me wrong about Baby Doe. I don't agree, but maybe you do.

The news story describes a visit with Baby Jane Doe, whose real name is Keri Lynn. Despite serious mental and physical impairments, she is doing well. She lives on Long Island, N.Y., with her parents and 1-year-old sister.

Keri Lynn was born with spina bifida, a genetic defect that, in her case, resulted in paralysis, incontinence, damaged kidneys and significant brain damage. Eight years ago, the question of whether the baby should receive aggressive medical care was the subject of a titanic legal battle pitting the federal government, various disability groups, Surgeon General C. Everett Koop and some right-to-life groups against the state of New York and the baby's parents.

The doctors said it was very likely that Keri Lynn would never be able to interact with other children and would live in great pain. Her parents, Dan and Linda, decided not to allow the doctors to perform surgery to drain fluid away from their baby's brain. They wanted conservative care—antibiotics but no surgery. And the doctors accepted their decision.

But a nurse did not. She tipped off an attorney active in the right-to-life movement that the baby was being allowed to die, and the Baby Jane Doe case began. The fight went all the way to the Supreme Court, which, in 1983, ruled in favor of the parents.

However, Congress subsequently did enact a law—the Child Abuse Amendments Act of 1984—that says that withholding care from a newborn who is not dead or imminently dying is child abuse. The law requires state child-welfare departments to monitor the care of newborns.

Much has changed in the years since Baby Jane Doe's case occupied the headlines. More has been learned about spina bifida. The physically impaired have fought hard to secure their rights. Disability is no longer so readily equated with a life not worth living.

Today, Keri Lynn is not in pain. She is able to interact with other people. Her parents and some health-care professionals think it may be many more years before she will require institutional care.

Eight years ago, I argued that Keri Lynn's parents should have the right to treat their daughter as they wished, within the boundaries of reasonable medical care. Nothing they did struck me as child neglect or abuse.

Has Keri Lynn proven me wrong? If surgery had been done, would her level of disability been less? Maybe.

In retrospect, there can be no denying that the level of misery predicted for Keri Lynn was way off the mark. And the battle over her care did much to change attitudes among doctors, nurses and the public about the prognosis faced by kids with spina bifida and other congenital birth defects.

But I still believe that the federal government was wrong to interfere in Keri Lynn's care. Her parents, while choosing a conservative course, never abandoned her and certainly never neglected her.

Laws that presuppose a lack of love between parents and children are lousy laws. The fact that state child-welfare departments have found no cases in which hospitals or parents have been guilty of abuse or neglect since Congress passed the 1984 Baby Doe law reinforces my view that it was and remains an unnecessary one. Telling neonatologists that they must aggressively treat premature and disabled infants is equivalent to passing laws requiring politicians to give long and windy speeches.

Keri Lynn is a reminder that medicine is an uncertain science. But, the battle over her medical care is also a reminder that, in the face of uncertainty, parents are in the best position to make hard choices among medical treatments of uncertain efficacy.

That is what her parents said then—and the love and care they have given Keri Lynn shows that letting parents decide is still best for children born with impairments now.

Collision of Cultures Should Not
Keep Boy from Walking

Six-year-old Kou Xiong was born in a Hmong refugee camp in Thailand. He had severely deformed clubfeet. But doctors at the camp had neither the skills nor the equipment necessary to undertake the surgery that would allow Kou to walk someday.

Even if they had been able to operate, Kou's parents, Houa Vue and Ger Xiong, would not have allowed it. They are deeply committed to animism, a spiritual outlook that views the efforts of doctors to repair congenital deformities as a violation of the will of the spirits.

County officials in Fresno, Calif., had to decide whether to force Kou to undergo corrective surgery.

Kou and his parents came to Fresno in 1989. When Kou began school, his teachers noticed his deformed feet. They were concerned that he had to use crutches or a wheelchair to get around and that he seemed to be in constant pain. They talked to Kou's parents, who said that their shaman had told them that Kou was born crippled in order to atone for the sins of his ancestors. He had to remain crippled, or evil spirits would wreak further havoc on Kou and the rest of the family.

The teachers took their concerns about Kou to Ernest Velasquez, Fresno County Social Services director. Velasquez had Kou examined by doctors from Valley Children's Hospital in Fresno and Shriners Hospital for Crippled Children in San Francisco. The doctors thought that Kou could walk without crutches if a series of operations was done to correct his clubfeet. They also said that without the operations, Kou would suffer irreparable damage to his hips and legs.

While Kou was being seen by the doctors, his parents had another child. The baby was born with a cleft palate—an affliction the parents took as a confirmation of what the shaman had said about the dangers of consulting doctors. They refused permission for Kou's surgery.

Velasquez sought a court order allowing the doctors to perform the operations. The district court issued an order allowing the surgery to be done, but Kou's parents' lawyer appealed.

Kou's case got all the way to the U.S. Supreme Court. On June 20, 1992, Supreme Court Justice Sandra Day O'Connor refused to set aside the lower court decision ordering the surgery.

But Kou's parents still refuse to give permission. They love Kou and are worried about the harm that the spirits will bring upon him, his siblings and the entire family if they allow the doctors to operate. Kou himself says that he does not want the surgery.

Kou's case has divided the Hmong community in northern California. Some argue that the state should respect the beliefs of the parents and not force surgery on Kou. Others argue that the animism of Kou's parents is an anachronism in the United States and that Kou will grow up bitter that he was allowed to remain permanently crippled because of his parents' old-fashioned beliefs.

Even though a court order exists allowing the surgery, no doctor will do it without Kou's parents' permission. Velasquez is not forcing the issue in the hope that Kou's parents eventually will change their minds.

If Kou had been born in the United States, federal laws governing the care of newborns would have required that the surgery be done, despite the objections of Kou's parents. Recently, a number of parents who are Christian Scientists have been convicted of manslaughter for refusing to obtain lifesaving medical care for their children.

While surgery in Kou's case is life-altering, not lifesaving, the operations still should be done, despite the fears of his parents. But Velasquez is right to try gentle persuasion rather than coercion with Kou and his family.

However, if Kou's parents do not change their minds, the county must find a doctor and a hospital willing to do the surgeries. The spiritual beliefs of Kou's parents should not be allowed to prevent him from walking.

Before Religion, Medicine Clash,
Protect the Kids

The other night, if you listened carefully, you could hear angels whispering in the halls of the Minnesota Capitol. The voices were those of children who died because their parents chose prayer over medicine.

They might have included Ian Lundman, an 11-year-old Minnesota boy who died from diabetes while his parents used spiritual healing instead of insulin. They might have been Shauntay Walker, a 4-year-old San Francisco girl who died in a coma from meningitis, or Ashley King, as 12-year-old Arizona girl who died in terrible pain from bone cancer; the girls' parents had refused to take them to a hospital.

These kids' spirits seemed to be asking legislators what they were going to do to prevent similar tragedies.

In Minnesota, as in many other states, the question of what to do when religion and medicine are in conflict is difficult to resolve. The Christian Science couple who provide spiritual healing for their sick baby, the Jehovah's Witness who opposes the use of blood or blood products for her daughter, the Hmong dad who believes that the shaman—not the surgeon—is his son's best hope for a cure are all acting from morally sound motives. They want to do what their consciences, cultures and hearts tell them is best for their children.

But public policy cannot be guided by religious or cultural belief systems when the lives of children are at stake. Medicine knows that kids ought to be immunized against measles, that a boy who has meningitis needs antibiotics and that a child with a blocked intestine needs surgery. The health interests of kids must take precedence over both parental rights and the freedom of religion. The question is how best to put these moral priorities into law.

In 1991, the South Dakota Legislature repealed the "shield" provision of the state's homicide statutes. You can no longer claim a religious right as a murder defense in South Dakota if your child dies because you did not seek timely medical care. Minnesota and other states could follow South Dakota's lead. Massachusetts followed in 1993.

But there is another legislative path that might do more to protect children than leaving parents open to homicide charges. Bills have been proposed in both the Minnesota House and Senate that call for the creation of a children's health-care mediator to be appointed by the state commissioner of health.

This person—most likely a public-health nurse—would be charged with reaching out to and communicating with various groups who prefer alternative healing practices over traditional medicine. The child-health mediator would educate parents about their duties and responsibilities in monitoring their children's health.

If parents believe their child is in a life-threatening situation or might suffer serious disability or disfigurement, they would have to report it immediately to the child-health monitor. Then, the monitor would visit the child, assess the medical circumstances and, if necessary, quickly get medical care for the child.

The idea behind this legislation is to use more of the carrot and less of the stick. The state would adopt a public-health model rather than a criminal-justice one for protecting the best interests of children. The legislation seeks to be proactive and cooperative rather than reactive and adversarial.

The health of children is more likely to be protected by working respectfully with parents to prevent harm rather than prosecuting them after a child has died.

Parents Thought Long and Hard
About "Experimental" Transplant

"Parenting is a difficult vocation." So began one of the most fascinating court opinions I have ever read, a deeply moving opinion issued by a Canadian judge.

David Arnot, a judge in the Provincial Court in North Battleford, Saskatchewan, faced a difficult decision. Should the parents of a young girl be allowed to refuse to consent to the only medical intervention capable of saving her life? He ruled that Francois and Leslie Paulette had the right to refuse permission for a liver transplant to be performed on their daughter, K'aila.

K'aila was born on June 13, 1989, near Fort Fitzgerald, Alberta. When she became sick six months later, her parents brought her to the Poundmaker Indian Reserve near Cut Knife, Saskatchewan. There she was seen by a traditional Indian healer. He said he could not help her and that she needed to see a physician.

K'aila was examined by a doctor who told her parents that she had been born with biliary atresia, a hereditary defect of the liver, for which there is no cure, except a liver transplant. Sixty-five percent of the children who receive a transplant survive at least five years.

K'aila's parents understood the death sentence that fate had handed their daughter. They also knew that a liver transplant was the only hope modern medicine could offer. The parents met with experts on transplantation. And they talked with two families whose children had had transplants.

They heard about the effects of the powerful drugs that transplant recipients must take daily. They worried about what the drugs might do to their daughter's development. They feared condemning her to a life of vulnerability to infections, medications and an uncertain long-term medical prognosis. They worried about her diminished quality of life.

They talked, they argued, they anguished. Finally, they told Dr. Calvin Stiller, one of Canada's most distinguished transplant surgeons, that they would not consent to surgery for K'aila.

The Department of Social Services was notified on the grounds that not doing the surgery might be an instance of child abuse. A trial was convened, during which three physicians testified that the decision to reject a transplant was reasonable; one argued that the surgery was essential.

Medical evidence about the efficacy of a liver transplant was never in doubt. But the judge was moved by more than medical facts and mathematical probabilities.

At one point, Leslie Paulette asked Judge Arnot, "Are these extraordinary medical procedures for prolongation of life the way society is supposed to deal with questions of life and death?"

The judge decided that the answer to Leslie Paulette's question was "no." In his ruling, he acknowledged that from a purely medical point of view, liver transplants have evolved into a standard medical therapy for biliary atresia. But, he said; other "components—practical, emotional, social and psychological," had to be taken into consideration.

Judge Arnot was convinced that the parents were trying to do what they believed was right for K'aila. He commented that no one could say the parents had not thought about what to do. He did not believe that saying no to a transplant represented "a clear case of rejection by the parents of the values society expects of thoughtful, caring parents for a terminally ill child." He refused to order the transplant and dismissed the case.

K'aila Paulette died in September of 1990. I know because her grandfather wrote to tell me so. He also said he believed the judge had done the right thing in refusing to order the transplant. He thought you should know that, too.

Doctor Obliged to Continue to Offer Help

A woman—I'll call her Eula Oleson—spent the last 14 of her 92 years in a nursing home in rural Minnesota.

For the past three years, she was confined to her bed by a variety of medical problems. The long stay in bed caused fluid to build up in her legs, leading to poor blood circulation.

Six months ago, Eula's legs began to turn black. The doctor who was caring for her said her only options were surgery on the veins in her legs, which almost certainly would not work, or amputation. Eula, still sharp and mentally alert, said no to both options. Her family backed her decision, knowing that saying no meant she would die.

The doctor agreed, grudgingly, to respect her wishes. Eula's legs continued to deteriorate. She began to suffer a lot of pain. Then, the doctor said that only amputation would prevent her death. Still she refused, so he prescribed morphine for her pain.

Eula got worse. She lost a great deal of weight. The doctors and nurses said she needed a feeding tube, but she refused. She only wanted her pain controlled.

Finally, about a month ago, Eula got to the point where she stopped asking for liquids. The morphine was controlling her pain, and she saw no need for food or water. The doctor came by nearly every day to offer her a feeding tube and intravenous fluids. Eula said no. In fact, she said that the doctor and the nurses should stop pestering her about food and water since she intended to die. They did stop.

Two weeks later, Eula Oleson died.

Did the doctor and the nursing staff do the right thing when they stopped offering food and water?

Recent controversies about the deaths of Nancy Cruzan and Helga Wanglie have focused public attention on the issue of whether it is right to withhold or withdraw food and water from a person who is incapable of making that choice.

But, at least as common—and equally troubling morally—is the question of what to do when a *competent* patient refuses food and water. Competent patients do have the right to refuse all forms of medical care, including food and water. They have this right even when that decision means they will die.

But, the choice to refuse food and water—as Eula Oleson did—raises this issue: How hard should health-care professionals try to change their patients' minds?

Is there ever a time when the offers of food and water should stop? When Eula Oleson told her doctor to stop bothering her about food and water, did she have that right, too? Or was it her doctor's duty to persist with the offers despite her instructions?

The line between badgering and offering is a thin one. But I think there is a duty to continue to offer medical treatment, including food and water, even to those who have emphatically refused it.

Eula Oleson, like you and me, has the right to say no. But she should also have had the right to change her mind right up to the moment of her death. As long as the doctor and the nursing staff did not hector or coerce her, as long as they made the offer of food and water at reasonable intervals—say every other day—they would not have violated her autonomy.

Patients such as Eula Oleson have the right to say no even to lifesaving medical treatments. But their health-care providers have the right—and the obligation—to make sure that patients mean what they say.

Hearing Families' Stories Leads
to Answers on Death Issues

The names are familiar—Quinlan, Brophy, Lawrance, Delio, Busalacchi, Rosebush, Cole, Wanglie, Mack, Amerman. These are the names of those Americans who pioneered a strange frontier, the boundaries of the right to die.

I have been invoking these names for many years in classrooms, lecture halls and articles as a kind of abstract shorthand—easy references to the key legal landmarks governing the right to say no more to medical technology. Those days are over.

The University of Minnesota Center for Biomedical Ethics organized a conference to examine issues around the right to die. In addition to the usual experts, some of the families who had lived through the legal battles, the protests and the media hounding were invited to speak. More than a dozen agreed to do so.

What they had to say about making life or death decisions for their spouses, sisters, sons and daughters, sisters- and brothers-in-law spoke volumes about how important it is to keep patient and family perspectives in the forefront of ethical debates about health care.

The stories of three family members were especially poignant. Joe and Julia Quinlan, Joyce, Christy and Joe Cruzan, and Pete Busalacchi made a convincing case that families must have primacy of decision-making authority when a patient is not capable of directing his or her medical care.

The Quinlans spoke with great dignity about their decision to remove a respirator from their daughter, Karen Ann. Before deciding on a course of action, they consulted their priest, their other children, friends and their hearts. They decided that no decision would be made unless the entire family agreed.

Ultimately, they decided that, knowing their daughter as they did, she would never want to remain a prisoner to technology that seemed to be a burden to her. The seven years that have passed since they won their court battle to allow a respirator to be stopped and Karen Ann died have not diminished their grief or confidence they did the right thing.

Jan. 11, 1993, was 10 years after a state patrolman found Nancy Beth Cruzan, then 25, lying unconscious and without any detectable signs of life by the side of her car on a rural Missouri road. Dec. 26, 1995 will be exactly five years since Nancy died.

She would have died sooner but for a battle between the Cruzan family and the Missouri Rehabilitation Center in Mount Vernon, Mo., over the removal of her feeding tube.

On Jan. 25, 1990, the U.S. Supreme Court ruled 5-4 that life-supporting technology, including food and fluids, could be removed from Nancy if there was clear and convincing evidence beyond what the family said that this is what she would have wanted.

Christy said the family was surprised. They could not understand why their views—the views of a close and loving father, mother and sister—would not be sufficient evidence of what Nancy would have wanted.

Joe Cruzan, still angry about the intrusion of so many strangers into his personal life, felt like the courts had "invited me to the Super Bowl, assigned me a seat in the last row of the bleachers while the game was played with my ball."

The Cruzans never wavered in their view that their fight to allow Nancy to die was what she would have wanted. Joe talked movingly about visiting her grave after all the press and protesters had left to tell his daughter that she "had just run ahead of the rest of the family but they would all catch up with her eventually."

Surely one test of who ought to have the authority to make decisions for incompetent patients is whether or not they will ever visit a grave or shed a tear once the lawyers and the cameras go away.

Pet Busalacchi was embroiled in a battle in the Missouri courts over the right to end life support for his daughter.

Pete wondered how anyone who had not taken her to soccer games, been at her birthday parties or taught her to drive in an empty parking lot could ever presume to have more legitimate authority about the course of her medical care than he does.

After listening to him and the other families—after hearing their expressions of love for those they have lost and outbursts of anger against strangers who felt no compunction about intruding into the most intimate of family matters—I think the only answer is that strangers have no place at the bedside.

Living Wills Might Not Make
a Difference, Study Finds

It has been months since a new federal law, the Patient Self-Determination Act, or PSDA, went into effect. The law guarantees that anyone admitted to a hospital, nursing home, hospice or home care program or who signs up with a health maintenance organization will get information on living wills.

The idea behind the PSDA is to prevent any more Karen Ann Quinlans, Nancy Cruzans or Helga Wanglies. By encouraging people to fill out living wills, to put in writing their wishes about what sort of medical care they would want should they become comatose or incompetent, the Congress hoped to end the tragic wrangles at the bedside among families, doctors, lawyers and administrators about when life-supporting treatment can be withdrawn or withheld.

The hope was admirable, but an article in the October 1, 1992 issue of the *Annals of Internal Medicine* shows that the PSDA is doomed to fail.

A team of researchers led by Dr. Lawrence Schneiderman of the University of California at San Diego decided to see whether living wills made any difference in the care of very sick patients. From 1987 to 1989, before the passage of the PSDA, they tracked 204 patients hospitalized at either the UCSD Medical Center or the Veterans Administration Medical Center in San Diego.

These patients all had serious, life-threatening illnesses such as heart disease, cancer and AIDS. Half were explicitly offered the chance to sign a living will, while the other half were not. Of those offered living wills, only two-thirds chose to fill them out. Of those who did, only two said they wanted aggressive treatment no matter what.

When patients completed a living will, a copy was put in their hospital records. In addition, an orange sticker was placed on the cover of their hospital chart to indicate they had a living will.

But, incredibly, Dr. Schneiderman and his colleagues found that filling out a living will had no bearing on the kind or degree of medical care these patients subsequently received.

There were no differences in the number of times those with living wills and those without them were actually resuscitated, had "do not resuscitate" orders written in their charts, or the numbers of days spent on respirators or attached to artificial feeding tubes.

Among those patients who died while in the study, those with living wills and those without them spent the same amount of time in the hospital and seemed to receive the same care. The cost of care for the two groups was "virtually identical—an average of approximately $19,000 per patient."

Living wills, which sound great in theory, had no influence in practice. One major reason was that few patients, even those who were clearly dying, actually lost the ability to make their wishes known. So there was no need to rely on their living will. Of the 204 very sick patients, only three fell into a state of dementia or permanent coma prior to their deaths.

The UCSD group draws an important conclusion from their research: "We find it hard to believe that any piece of paper, however artfully designed, will suffice as a satisfactory means of doctor-patient communication."

Despite the dreams of lawyers and legislators, there is no substitute for talk when the subject is medical care for serious illness.

The only way to prevent future Karen Ann Quinlans, Nancy Cruzans or Helga Wanglies is to make sure that we have a health care system that insists that health care providers and patients talk openly and freely and that provides them with the financial incentives and time to do so.

CHAPTER 5
DEFINING DEATH, EUTHANASIA
AND THE RIGHT TO DIE

If Mother Dies, Should Her Fetus Live On?

Is it morally right to keep a dead woman who is pregnant attached to life support machines in order to let her fetus live? A case in California shows that such a question is not hypothetical.

Trisha Marshall died of a gunshot wound to the head on April 21, 1993 while 17 weeks pregnant. David Smith, the father, asked hospital officials to do whatever they could to save the fetus. Marshall's body was kept on life support machines at Highland hospital in Oakland in the hope that her fetus would develop to the point where it could live.

On Aug. 4, a 4-pound, 15-ounce baby boy was delivered four weeks prematurely by Caesarean section. Dr. Richard Fulroth, who headed the team that delivered the child, called him "a miracle baby."

Some, such as the Smith family, see the situation as offering no choice—if you can save the child by maintaining the mother's corpse, doctors must try. But the idea of maintaining a corpse to rescue a child strikes some as morally abhorrent.

Doubts about the morality of using a cadaver to allow a fetus to develop were much in evidence last year in Germany in a similar case, that of the "Erlanger baby."

The storm of ethical debate that greeted the decision to try and save this fetus is recounted in a fascinating article by Christoph Anstotz in the journal *Bioethics*.

On Oct. 5, 1992, a young woman named Marion Ploch was driving home from her job as a dental assistant. Somehow, she lost control of her car and hit a tree at high speed. Medical help arrived quickly.

Within 15 minutes, she had been transported by helicopter to the university hospital in the Southern German city of Erlanger. She had suffered massive head injuries in the crash.

Her parents were told their daughter had no hope of recovery. They were also told that she was 13 weeks pregnant. No one knew who the father was.

Some of the doctors asked about Ploch's status as an organ donor. Others, however, thought that there might be a chance of saving the fetus if Marion was kept on artificial life support. The parents were not certain what to do.

On Oct. 8, the doctors declared Ploch dead but did not discontinue her life support. A day later, her parents, still uncertain about what to do, spoke with a reporter from a large German newspaper, *Bild-Zeitung*. The reporter called the hospital to ask what the doctors planned to do. A committee was convened, and on Oct. 11 Ploch's parents and doctors agreed to try and continue the pregnancy until the fetus could be delivered safety by Cesarean section.

Once the decision had been made, the doctors were vigorous in defense of it. The assistant medical director told the press, "There really isn't any question whether it should be tried or not ... We don't see any ethical reason simply to let the embryo die."

The hospital's director, Franz Paul Gall, agreed, saying, "The child's right to live demands also the use of modern and technological aids."

But, as Anstotz notes in his article, many did not agree with the decision of the parents and the doctors. Opposition to the decision made for some might strange bedfellows.

Some doctors condemned the decision to maintain Ploch's body as a "shameless human experiment ... a perversion of the oath of Hippocrates." The left-wing environmental Green Party organized a petition drive and quickly gathered 7,000 signatures that they sent to the Ministry of Justice demanding an immediate halt to "the human experiment."

Hanna Wolf, spokeswoman for women's affairs in the German Parliament, said the decision to try to bring Ploch's baby to term "is a scandal and inhuman. The mother is degraded to nutrient fluid, disposable after use." Many other feminists and academics agreed that keeping a woman artificially alive was disrespectful of the dignity of the deceased mother.

Feminist critics and environmentalists were joined by a chorus of theologians. The Catholic chaplain at the hospital, Rainer Denkler, said, "I cannot share in the decision to respirate and nourish a brain-dead young woman for several months in order to make possible the birth of a 14-week-old embryo."

Another prominent Catholic theologian argued that "to allow nature to take its course in this matter [and turn off the machines] cannot be morally equivalent to a direct killing of human life in the event of an abortion."

A well-known Protestant theologian proclaimed that "the right of the intact living and dying includes the right to a dignified burial, and it is to be accepted that it is the destiny of mother and child to die."

About the strongest praise any theologians and religious leaders could muster for the effort was that it was not "ethically careless." The public apparently had its doubts too. In a newspaper telephone poll taken late in 1992 asking "Is it right for a dead woman to have a child?" 33,436 respondents said no, as against 7,302 who said yes.

It is not clear why there was so much opposition in Germany to the decision to try to rescue Ploch's fetus and so little in the United States over the effort to save Trisha Marshall's. The Marshall case was a success. The effort to save the Erlanger baby failed. The fetus was born dead on Nov. 16, 1992. But the criticism started long before the outcome of the rescue attempt was known.

Granted, trying to rescue a fetus in the body of a woman who has died is an experiment. Not all families will choose this course of action. But is it really such a morally heinous thing to do to use a dead body to try to preserve the life of a fetus, when the closest next-of-kin give their consent to the rescue effort?

Surely, it is not unreasonable to think in the absence of any evidence to the contrary that a mother would want an effort to be made to save her fetus. And if a husband, parents or other family members decide that the attempt to save the fetus is the right thing to do, it is hard to see why others would say that maintaining the body on machines to allow the fetus to develop is disrespectful to the mother.

Using a cadaver to save the life of a developing fetus is risky, unusual and maybe even macabre. But it is not immoral.

We Can't Blur Line Between
Life and Death

Theresa Ann Campo Pearson did not have a very long life. When she died in April, 1992, she was only 10 days old. Despite her short life, she became the center of a very strange, sad and wrenching ethical controversy.

Theresa died because her brain had failed to form. She had anencephaly, a condition in which only the brain stem, located at the top of the spinal cord, is present. Her parents wanted her to be an organ donor. The courts said no.

It seems strange that the parents did not get their way. Why not allow donation when every day in North America a baby dies because there is no heart, lung or liver available for transplantation? Yet, the courts had no choice but to rule the way they did.

Anencephaly is best described as completely "unabling," not disabling. Children such as Theresa, born with anencephaly, cannot think, feel, sense or be aware of the world. Many are stillborn. The majority of the rest are dead within days. A mere handful live for a few weeks.

Theresa's parents, Laura Campo and Justin Pearson, knew all this. But, rather than abort the pregnancy, they chose to have their baby. In fact, the baby was born by Caesarean section, at least partly in the hope that it would be born alive, thereby making organ donation possible. Laura and Justin fervently wanted something good to come from their personal tragedy.

But, when Theresa died at Broward General Medical Center in Fort Lauderdale, Fla., no organs were taken. Two Florida courts had ruled that the baby could not be used as a source of organs unless she was brain dead. And Theresa Ann Campo Pearson was never pronounced brain dead.

Brain death refers to a situation in which the brain has irreversibly lost all function, all activity. Babies born with anencephaly have some brain function in their brain stem. So, while they cannot think or feel, they are alive.

Doctors can tell with certainty in adults when brain death occurs. But, current technology cannot accurately measure brain activity in a tiny bit of brain in an infant. A child like Theresa cannot be diagnosed as brain dead because the amount of brain cells she had are too small to accurately measure.

By Florida law—and the law in more than 40 other states—only those persons declared brain dead can donate organs. The courts of Florida had no other option than to deny the request for organ donation. Ironically, the very condition that took Theresa's life made it impossible for the doctors to tell whether she was dead in the way that the law requires for organ donation to take place.

One obvious solution is to change the law. States could decide that organs could be removed from either those who are brain dead or babies who are born with anencephaly. Or, the definition of death could be rewritten to say that death occurs either when the brain has totally ceased to function or if a baby is born anencephalic.

Either change appears plausible. But neither should be made.

If people believe that medicine will fudge the line between life and death in order to get organs for transplant, they will become even more skeptical about the whole field of organ donation. Many now refuse to check off their driver's license donation box or carry a donor card because they worry that if they are known to be potential organ donors, they will not be aggressively treated at the hospital. Changing the definition of death to include anencephaly will only exacerbate those fears.

What Can Be Worse Than Death?
Many Say Suffering, Dependence

What frightens you the most about becoming seriously ill? What do you think of when you hear of a relative, friend or celebrity stricken by cancer, heart disease or Alzheimer's?

Maybe you think most people would say dying. But, according to a recent study by a team of researchers at the University of Washington in Seattle, many of us think there are many situations that are worse than death.

Unfortunately, our health care system is not doing what it should to attend to these concerns. Robert Pearlman, a physician specializing in geriatric care at the Seattle Veterans Health Center, and a group of his colleagues published a fascinating study on patient assessments of states worse than death in the *Journal of Clinical Ethics*.

Pearlman's group conducted in-depth, structured interviews with 56 adults. These were not just folks off the street. They were people who had stared death squarely in the face. Some of those interviewed had AIDS. Some had spent time in a coma following a heart attack. Eight had a terminal illness such as cancer.

The researchers asked this group under what circumstances they thought it might be preferable to be dead rather than alive. The answers they gave are fascinating, disturbing and illuminating about changes that are long overdue in our health care system.

- Ninety-six percent said that they felt it would be worse to be kept alive under hopeless circumstances, when "death is just outside the front door," than it would be to actually die.
- Eighty-two percent believed that the total loss of independence would be worse than death. They found the prospect of their bodies becoming incapacitated, being left by disease or injury unable to feed, dress or clothe themselves more frightening than the prospect of death.
- Seventy-nine percent said they hated the idea of dying in a strange place more than the idea of death itself.
- And 73 percent were so averse to a life of unremitting pain and suffering that they would rather be dead.

How well is medicine doing in helping patients cope with these concerns? To say lousy would be a generous assessment. Doctors and nurses spend far too much time manipulating technology and too little talking to their seriously ill patients about their hopes, fears and concerns.

As Pearlman and his colleagues note, the concerns expressed by those they interviewed "are not the usual subject matter for clinician-patient discussions."

Not only are the subjects of hope, independence and setting of death rarely discussed, a survey in the *Annals of Internal Medicine* conducted by a team of doctors headed by Jamie Von Roenn of the Northwestern University Medical School in Chicago indicates that there is much too high a chance that those who fear pain and suffering more than death have reason to worry.

Von Roenn and his team asked 897 doctors—including surgeons, hematologists, oncologists, internists and radiologists—who care for patients with cancer about the treatment of pain in those patients.

Nearly nine in 10 of the doctors said they think that the majority of cancer patients do not get adequate medication for pain control. Only 51 percent of the cancer specialists thought that the pain control in the institutions where they practice is good or very good.

Why? Three-fourths thought that inadequate efforts to assess pain in patients was the single most important obstacle to good pain management. Other major barriers to the treatment of pain are the reluctance of some doctors to prescribe narcotic drugs due to worries about side effects or addictions; patient reluctance to say they are in pain; and patient fears about the side effects of pain-relieving drugs, such as becoming incoherent or overly tired.

Von Roenn and his associates think a revolution in the training of physicians and nurses in pain management is in order. Those who treat patients with cancer and other serious illnesses need to know how to properly assess pain in their patients. They also need to reassure patients that complaints about pain do not mean they are "bad" patients.

And physicians and patients need to learn to talk to one another about how to use the drugs that are available in ways that permit pain to be controlled with tolerable side effects.

For many of us, there are things in life that are worse than death. For too many who practice in the health care field, the only thing to worry about is death. Unless our health care system begins to take hope, independence, comfort and pain more seriously there is every reason to fear that the public will insist upon laws and legislation that let those who are seriously ill choose death as the lesser evil.

Euthanasia Essay Should
Have Been Killed

A friend called me the other day to ask if I had seen either the March 2 or March 23, 1992 editions of *Newsweek* magazine. "No," I said, "I hadn't." "Go find them," he said. "You won't believe your eyes."

I did. And he was right—I didn't. What I found in the magazine made me furious. It should make you furious, too.

On March 2, the editors of *Newsweek* saw fit to print a vicious screed by someone named Katie Letcher Lyle. Lyle, who is identified as a free-lance writer and a volunteer on three boards advocating on behalf of the handicapped, penned an essay in which she said that mentally retarded people would be better off dead.

She arrived at this despicable conclusion by drawing an analogy between the decision she made to euthanize her 16-year-old cat, which was dying of cancer, and the plight of the severely retarded who face life in overcrowded state institutions or on the cruel streets.

Lyle gave other reasons beyond veterinary ethics for wanting to kill the retarded. She notes that paying the costs of caring for the retarded and mentally ill is very burdensome to the American taxpayer. She favors knocking off these useless, unhappy leeches before the national debt gets any bigger.

The fact that a major news magazine saw fit to print such utter bilge and then devoted space later in its letters section to readers' arguments, merits a bit more scorn than this inexcusable breach of media ethics has so far elicited.

What was *Newsweek* thinking when it chose to publish Lyle's essay? Can we now look forward to future opinion pieces on the need to exterminate the Jews before they ruin the racial purity of the nation? Will *Newsweek* be filling its pages with editorials and letters from those who believe that everyone with HIV ought to be killed in order to reduce health-care costs?

Newsweek appears to have been able to publish Lyle's call to return to the heyday of the Third Reich without much of a peep from its media brethren. Is this because the targets of Lyle's benevolent euthanasia policies are the retarded and the mentally ill—groups who lack much of a political lobby and buy few magazines?

The publication of an essay equating human beings with cats and calling for euthanasia in the name of cost-containment serves as a timely reminder that the vulnerable in our society are dependent on the moral vigilance of others to defend their rights. When a respected publication sees fit to put in print an essay that demeans, dehumanizes and imperils the helpless by calling for their murder, it is time to rethink our media as well as our medial ethics.

Dr. Jack's Back, and This Guy is Really Scary

Freddy, the notorious star of the slasher genre, may finally be dead, but Dr. Jack is back again.

Despite an Oakland County, Mich., court order prohibiting him from using his "suicide machine," Dr. Jack Kevorkian thumbed his nose at the judicial system and helped two more Michigan women kill themselves on October 30, 1991.

He had assisted in the death last year of another woman, Janet Adkins, who came to Michigan from Oregon to commit suicide when she became despondent upon learning that she had Alzheimer's disease.

Kevorkian aided the suicides of Sherry Miller, 43, of Roseville, Mich., who had a severe case of multiple sclerosis, and Marjorie Wantz, 58, of Sodus, Mich. Wantz suffered from a painful but not immediately life-threatening condition known as pelvic adhesions. Neither woman was terminally ill. Both had been asking Kevorkian to help them die for years.

Wantz died using the latest model of Kevorkian's machine. Miller inhaled carbon monoxide through a mask supplied by Kevorkian. Both died in the setting Kevorkian has come to favor—a state park.

There are many who said Kevorkian did not kill anyone. He merely assisted. This absurd line of argument so befuddled Michigan's courts that they rejected a murder charge in the death of Janet Adkins on the grounds that Adkins killed herself by throwing the switch on the suicide machine.

Baloney!

Kevorkian built the machines that killed Adkins and Wantz. He has spent the past few years looking for people to use them. He was present when all three women died. He helped attach them to their devices of death. And he supplied the instructions on how to use them. Flicking a switch is the end of a chain of events that points right to Kevorkian.

The legal system of Michigan should be summarily disbarred if it cannot make a murder charge stick under these circumstances. The important question is not whether Kevorkian killed these women, but whether what he did was morally right. And it wasn't.

The women who died needed no medical assistance if they wanted to kill themselves. They were competent women who could have used any of a number of methods to end their lives. It appears the only reason they sought out Kevorkian is that they wanted their deaths to be clean, neat and quick. They wanted someone else to do what they could not bring themselves to do.

Those are not good enough reasons for doctors to help people commit suicide or for our society to allow them to do so. Our laws should make suicide hard, not easy. Suicide and assisting in a suicide should be messy, disturbing, troubling, trying and difficult.

Another reason Kevorkian's actions are immoral is that he is in no position to serve as a plausible arbiter of death. This is a man who has been a tireless advocate for euthanasia. He is the wrong man to counsel anyone whose illness, pain and disability lead them to think about killing themselves. These people need to talk to a doctor who believes suicide is a bad idea—not a good one.

Kevorkian has shown himself to be a clear and present danger. He has now helped many kill themselves and has yet to face a day in jail for it.

America has worked itself into a frenzy over the death of one person who got AIDS from a health-care professional. Where's the moral outrage over a doctor who deliberately assists in the suicides of many people?

Courtroom Wrong Site to "Settle"
National Debate on Euthanasia

Americans seem congenitally unable to learn from the past. The latest demonstration of our inability to glance backward in our constant struggle to move forward took place in a Michigan courtroom.

Jack Kevorkian, ex-pathologist, self-appointed visionary and artiste extraordinaire (whose aesthetic muse, if you look at his bizarro paintings, must be the Cryptmaster from HBO's "Tales From the Crypt"), finally got his day in court.

Kevorkian and his histrionic lawyer/thespian sidekick, Geoffrey Fieger, mewed for months that they wanted a Michigan court to examine the good doctor's actions in using carbon monoxide gas to poison Thomas Hyde. Hyde was afflicted with a terrible, degenerative disease. He sought Kevorkian's irreversible form of relief for suffering and pain.

But, after their chance to test the legality of Michigan's statute that prohibits assisted suicide. Kevorkian and his bulldog attorney turned things into a sad joke. While brave outside the courtroom, the Kevorkian defense turned wimpy once inside. Most of the trial consisted of a hunt for legal technicalities that might get Kevorkian off the hook.

The case was wrongly brought, Kevorkian's attorney whined, because Hyde did not die near Detroit but nearby in Oakland County. The technical language of the Michigan law did not apply to Kevorkian's actions with respect to Hyde because the doctor merely intended to alleviate his suffering. Michigan law exempts from prosecution deaths that occur in the course of physician attempts to use high doses of pain-relieving drugs.

Carbon monoxide gas, which Kevorkian used to help Hyde die, hardly fits the category of a pain-relieving drug. Still, this escape clause was seized upon with fervor by a legal team suddenly committed to finding any available loophole through which they and their client might slither away.

"What did the trial mean?" the media kept asking. "What was its significance?" Are these people kidding? Unless they were raised as one of the various innocents who composed the Brady bunch, these representatives of the Fourth Estate must know that the trial represented Kevorkian's best chance to claim victory for his particularly zany approach to euthanasia.

A conviction only meant appeals, more histrionics and, ultimately, a plea of victimization by a cruel judiciary indifferent to the pain and suffering endured by those Kevorkian has killed. A verdict of not guilty would only have meant a claim of complete vindication for Dr. K. The outcome of the trial never mattered—Kevorkian would come away a winner whatever the outcome.

Which brings me back to the issue of ignoring the past. For more than 20 years this nation has had to live with the consequences of a judicial resolution to a divisive social issue—abortion. When Roe vs. Wade was issued in 1973, it became the battleground over which the pro- and anti- forces fought for their believes.

Appointments to the Supreme Court now hinge on where one stands on that decision. Decisions about reproduction and procreation have become matters for judges, civil rights organizations and all manner of courtroom devotees.

I support Roe vs. Wade. I think the legal reasoning in the case was fundamentally sound. But I regret that the abortion controversy ended in a courtroom. The judicial resolution was not enough to bring social consensus on the subject.

Physician-assisted suicide—or, for that matter, assisted suicide—is, like abortion, an issue that should be decided by the American people and their legislators, not courts.

Surely the courts must remain on guard to protect against violations of fundamental, constitutional rights. Tyrannical majorities cannot be allowed to deprive others of their liberty and freedom. But courts are ill-suited to settle difficult and divisive social issues. Political and legislative resolutions are also needed.

The trial of Dr. Kevorkian is not our decade's version of the Scopes trial. It represents a tiny blip in the evolving national debate about euthanasia and assisted suicide. If we don't realize the need for political answers to what are vexing moral questions, we condemn ourselves and our children to the kind of social fractiousness and zealotry that have torn this nation apart ever since another court "resolved" the abortion issue.

Doctor Stayed Involved in Life,
Not Suicide

Timothy Quill, a staff physician at the Genesee Hospital in Rochester, N.Y., tells an incredibly sad and disturbing story about one of his patients in the March 7, 1991 issue of the *New England Journal of Medicine*. The story is sad because it ends with the death of Quill's patient; it is troubling because Quill prescribed the sleeping pills that his patient used to kill herself.

Quill's story comes hard on the heels of another widely discussed assisted suicide: that of Janet Adkins. She died in June in a trailer park near Detroit while attached to a machine built by Dr. Jack Kevorkian.

I am convinced that what Kevorkian did in helping Janet Adkins die is completely immoral. Yet, I do not believe that Quill acted unethically.

In order to understand why, you need to know more about what happened to Quill's patient, Diane. Quill diagnosed Diane, 45, as having acute myelomonocytic leukemia—a fatal form of cancer. When he told her she had leukemia, he said it could be treated by chemotherapy or by a bone-marrow transplant.

Diane considered the odds: about a 25 percent chance of survival. She thought about the side effects of the treatments, which are almost always awful and are sometimes fatal themselves. She rejected both forms of treatment.

Quill tried hard to talk Diane into accepting treatment. He knew her well, knew that she already had beaten vaginal cancer, depression and alcoholism, knew of her recent success in her marriage, her work and her artistic pursuits. He argued that the odds were not that bad, that she should try to beat the leukemia. But Diane said no.

Neither Diane's family nor Quill could change her mind. Knowing that without treatment Diane's condition would rapidly deteriorate, Quill arranged for home hospice care.

During the next few weeks, Diane did not change her mind about refusing treatment. She did, however, ask Quill how she could take her own life if the process of her dying became unbearable.

Quill understood her fear and her need to remain in control. He assured her that he would do all he could to control her pain. But he also felt obligated to tell her about the Hemlock Society, an organization he knew could provide her with information about suicide.

About a week later, Diane asked for barbiturates to help her sleep. Quill understood that she was having trouble sleeping, but he also knew that she wanted the pills in case she decided to kill herself. He wrote the prescription. And Diane filled it.

Several months later, after long bouts of bone pain, weakness, fatigue and fever, and knowing that her death was imminent, Diane killed herself by taking a deliberate overdose of the pills.

Both Jack Kevorkian and Timothy Quill were involved in assisting in a suicide. But ethically, the two have nothing in common. Kevorkian did not know Janet Adkins prior to attaching her to his homemade suicide device. Quill had known Diane both as a patient and a friend for many years prior to her death. Kevorkian scoured the country looking for someone upon whom he could use his machine. Quill did all that he could to get his patient to choose life, not death.

Kevorkian helped a woman to die who was questionably competent, was in no pain and who was not terminally ill; Quill wrote a prescription for sleeping pills for a terminally ill, competent woman who was in a great deal of pain. Kevorkian personally hitched Janet Adkins to a machine that he himself had built, promoted and fervently hoped someone would use; Quill fervently hoped he could help manage Diane's suffering so that she would never choose to end her life.

Kevorkian and Quill both played a role in the death of one of their patients. But Kevorkian directly assisted in the death of a person who was nearly a complete stranger to him, from motives that were, at best, suspect. Quill did what he could to persuade his patient to struggle on in the face of a painful illness. When that battle was lost, he confined his participation in her death to the writing of a prescription. Quill conducted himself ethically. Kevorkian did not.

This is Living? Or, Why Bother to Save Your Brain?

The fate of my head has been on my mind in recent days. I've been trying to decide what to do when the day comes when I no longer have any use for the old noggin.

When the grim reaper makes his presence known to me, should I arrange to have my head lopped off and frozen in a tank of liquid nitrogen? This course of action might create the possibility that in the future a kindly doctor will decide to de-ice the thing, attach it to a handy mechanical body, revivify the resulting hybrid and then sit down with my cranium in order to better understand the dangers that co-dependency, MTV and Donald Trump posed to 20th century humankind.

Imagine, if this scenario actually worked, my head would enjoy an endless future of writing articles, flossing and visits to the hairstylist.

There is a more altruistic route available to me as I mull the fate of my pate. I might choose to spare the healers of tomorrow the burden of dealing with my defrosting dome, and will my head—or at least its contents—to science. The Brain Tissue Resource Center at McLean Hospital in Belmont, Mass., thoughtfully mailed me a pamphlet to let me know that they are keenly interested in my brain, but only on the condition that I not be alive to present it to them.

The scientists point out that there is "enormous potential in postmortem human brain research ... in understanding severe neurologic and psychiatric disorders" but that progress is "being delayed because of a scarcity of brain tissue donors."

My inspiration concerning the option of flash-freezing my noodle comes from the lawsuit that Thomas Donaldson, a 46-year-old mathematician from Sunnyside, Calif., filed with the California attorney general's office. Donaldson has a brain tumor that his doctors believe stands a good chance of killing him. He is suing in order to guarantee that as the time of his demise draws nigh he will have the right to have his head surgically removed, frozen and stored at the Alcor Life Extension Foundation, a cryonics society based in Riverside, Calif.

Donaldson is motivated by ego, not altruism. His hope is that medical science will someday figure out how to cure his tumor and will then attach his head to a handy body. If he waits, however, until the tumor kills him, he fears there may not be enough brain tissue left for the doctors of tomorrow to defrost.

There is a bitter irony in my receipt of a request for brain tissue donation at the same time that Donaldson went to court to secure his inalienable right to alienate himself from his head. If I refuse to donate my brain to science, how will the doctors of tomorrow learn enough about diseases of the brain to defrost Thomas Donaldson's head and restore it to a chatty, amiable state?

On the other hand, why should I play the sap so that Donaldson can become a living fossil for the denizens of 25th century Earth? Would it not be smarter for me to encourage Donaldson to assign his head for post-mortem research and development? I can then prepare my own noggin for an enviable future as the ultimate talk show guest on whatever passes for Oprah or Donahue in the centuries to come.

Actually, if you use your head in the here and now, you would realize that it might not be such an attractive thing to find your head awake and refreshed 200 or 300 years after the rest of you had turned to dust. After all, you would be a crushing bore at cocktail parties bandying about names such as Prince, Madonna, Gerald Ford and Geraldo Rivera.

And as soon as you got your head on straight you would be confronted with a whopping medical bill from the doctors who rekindled your cranium. Even if medical costs only go up 5 percent a year, by 2400 you'll be talking some serious bucks.

Forget immortality. It is simply not what it is cracked up to be once you take a closer look. At best, Thomas Donaldson's head will wind up a couple of hundred years from now faced with the problem of balancing a very old checkbook.

If you want to do something really worthwhile with your head, donate it to medical science.

CHAPTER 6
AIDS, EPIDEMICS, PUBLIC HEALTH AND POPULATION

Make a Leap of Faith?
It's an AIDS Dilemma

AIDS hysteria infected Minnesota in June of 1991, after two Twin Cities physicians, Dr. Philip Benson and Dr. Richard Duff, admitted that they had been practicing medicine while knowing that they were HIV-positive—but without telling their patients.

Hardly anyone managed to escape the terrible consequences of the outbreak: anger, fear, outrage, anxiety and panic. Later in the week, other outbreaks were reported in Hershey, Pa., and South Florida as new cases of HIV-positive physicians went public.

When HIV gets into a person's cells, little can be done. When AIDS hysteria erupts, much more can and must be done.

First, we must understand the causes of AIDS hysteria. After all, Americans have been the targets of a nearly decade-long AIDS public-education campaign involving government at every level, the media, health-care professionals, AIDS activists, educational associations and religious groups.

Everyone from C. Everett Koop to Liz Taylor to Jon Bon Jovi has repeated the mantra of prevention: The best way to prevent AIDS is to avoid intravenous drug use and unprotected sexual intercourse. The public has been told that the only way to get the virus is by blood or fluid contact. And, time and time again, our radios, TVs and newspapers have reminded us that the chance of contracting AIDS from a single instance of blood or bodily fluid exchange is tiny—far less than the chance of being murdered, killed in an automobile or airplane accident, or dying from a firearms accident.

Why do all the efforts at education go for naught in the face of HIV-positive health-care providers? The reason is that when a doctor has AIDS, he or she is seen as posing a risk to people who normally do not worry about the disease. The reaction when a doctor or dentist has AIDS is so strong because, for almost a decade, Americans have been content to ghettoize AIDS. Once it became clear that you do not get AIDS from toilet seats, sneezing or food, and once the predicted breakout from heterosexual contact failed to materialize, AIDS, for most Americans, became a disease for others to worry about: the poor, minorities, the addicted and the sexually deviant.

The education has been going in one ear and out the other because most Americans believe they are not at risk—until confronted with the reality of an HIV-infected doctor, dentist or nurse.

The hysteria on display this week is not based on irrationality or ignorance. It is the anguish mainstream America feels when it finds itself at risk.

If risk to mainstream America is the cause of the outbreak, then what are the cures? Are organized medicine and our governments ready to deal with the reality of HIV-infected health-care workers?

Benson announced at a June 15, 1991 press conference that he had practiced family medicine at the Palen Clinic and Riverside Medical Center in Minneapolis for the past year, all the time knowing that he was HIV-positive. Duff went public a few days later. Both said they had cared for patients while HIV-positive with the full knowledge of Minnesota's Department of Health and Board of Medical Examiners. Incredibly, Benson practiced from May 1990 to February 1991 with a serious bacterial infection that caused fluid to ooze from open sores on his hands. Benson said he had taken care to glove and double-glove while doing prenatal exams, rectal exams, vaginal exams and deliveries of babies. State officials were satisfied that both Benson and Duff should have been allowed to care for patients as long as they avoided surgery or other procedures inside their patients with sharp objects.

Officials in Minnesota, as in other states, felt no obligation to make public the name of either doctor. Nor did they insist that the doctors tell their patients they were HIV-positive. They felt that as long as the risks of infection were tiny or nonexistent, privacy should hold sway over mandatory disclosure. But there are no formal guidelines governing what should be done when a doctor or nurse is HIV-positive. The federal government has promised action, but none has been forthcoming.

Benson's announcement that he had continued delivery babies with open sores on his hands, knowing that he was HIV-positive, was the Ground Zero of AIDS hysteria in Minnesota. A decade's worth of public education evaporated in an instant.

Officials of Minnesota's health department and Board of Medical Examiners had been powerless to stop Benson because they apparently did not know what he was doing. The best the health department could do was to undertake a "look-back" at the records of all his patients to see which ones had been in blood or fluid contact with him, in order to notify them that they should consider being tested for HIV.

In all, 328 letters were sent under Benson's name urging testing; more than 280 people have come in to the University of Minnesota Hospital. Many of those who arrived for their "anonymous" tests were greeted by a swarm of television cameras and reporters who seemed less interested in protecting their anonymity than in finding someone who would curse the day they ever met Benson.

Have government and organized medicine properly discharged their responsibilities to the public?

In the case of Duff, they did. Allowing Duff to continue his practice without telling his patients that he had the AIDS virus makes sense because he did nothing that posed a risk to any of them.

Matters are very different with respect to Benson. Benson should not have been delivering babies or doing rectal exams with open, festering sores on his hands—AIDS or no AIDS, gloves or no gloves. As soon as the Board of Medical Examiners found out about his bacterial infection, he should have immediately been suspended from all patient contact. But the board did not know what he was doing. And that is not acceptable.

AIDS poses the tiniest of risks where physicians, nurses or dentists are the source. You are more at risk of dying while driving to see a surgeon who is HIV-positive than you are of dying as a result of getting the virus from that surgeon. Still, no HIV-infected doctor, dentist or nurse should be allowed to have blood or fluid contact with a patient without the patient's knowledge and consent. Tiny risks are still risks, and patients have the right to know about them.

Patients who will come in blood or bodily fluid contact with their physicians have a right to known whether they are HIV-positive. While there is no need for general testing of all workers, government has the obligation to make sure that physicians, dentists and nurses who have blood or fluid contact with patients undergo mandatory, periodic testing to determine their HIV status and to detect any other communicable diseases.

But mandatory testing and the duty to disclose cut both ways. Doctors, dentists and nurses who come into contact with the blood or bodily fluids of patients have every right to require them to consent to testing for HIV and other communicable diseases. And though they have no right to deny care, they do have a right to know the results of those tests.

Privacy must yield to safety at the bedside.

Ban Shows Bias Against
All AIDS Victims

Every so often, a public-policy decision is made that is so dumb, so knuckleheaded, so out of touch with the facts that even in the daily parade of oddities that pass for government policy, the decision stands out. Such is the nature of the federal government's decision to retain its immigration ban against those who are infected with the AIDS virus.

I know what you're thinking: Here comes another bleeding-heart broadside against any law or policy that inhibits the rights of those who have AIDS. Isn't the Bush administration [1991] right to worry about the costs associated with treating AIDS, you may ask? It is one thing to open our doors to those yearning to be free. It's quite another to pay the bill for treating immigrants with AIDS.

Indeed, the administration cites the high costs associated with the medical treatment of AIDS as its primary rationale for maintaining the ban. But let's allow a little reality to cloud this argument. Suppose you live in Haiti, the Netherlands, Brazil, Tanzania or Thailand and you found out you had AIDS. Let's also suppose you are poor. Would your first response be to book a flight to the States?

Well, think about it. What is the reality of health care for the poor in American today? Is it such as to make those in other lands, even those who are desperately poor, pull up stakes and relocate here? Hardly.

The hospitals that bear the brunt of caring for the poor—public facilities in large cities—are in a state of near collapse. The quality of care for those on Medicaid or who lack insurance in New York, Los Angeles, Detroit, Houston, Miami and New Orleans is not likely to attract too many foreigners with AIDS.

Our urban hospitals, as any first-year resident who works in one will tell you, cannot adequately care for those currently seeking care. Waiting lists are long, emergency rooms are crowded, babies who are HIV positive languish in neonatal nurseries and overcrowding is often so bad that acutely ill patients lie in beds in the corridors.

Faced with a diagnosis of AIDS, is it really likely that a foreigner's first response will be to come here in order to join the line of 50 million Americans who have inadequate insurance or the 37 million who have none?

But the conceit that we will have to beat back hordes of AIDS-infected immigrants from our shores does not end with the failure to touch base with the misery that is health care for the poor in our nation. The ban misses the psychological realities of terminal illness.

If you have AIDS, the chances are especially good that you will want to stay in your own home. If you are very sick or dying, the chances are good that you will want to stay close to those who know and love you rather than travel to a foreign land to live out your remaining days in a strange setting.

If immigration by AIDS victims were a real problem, the countries of western Europe, Scandinavia and Canada, which all have better health-care services for the poor than we do, would be swamped by people with AIDS trying to sneak across their borders. They aren't. Given the state of our health care system for the poor, we won't be, either.

Like Critic, Rethink Opposition to
Needle Exchange Programs

I have long had strong reservations about the wisdom of needle exchange programs aimed at controlling the spread of AIDS among addicts.

My doubts have nothing to do with a failure to understand the enormity of the problem. Nearly a third of all AIDS cases in the United States are the result of needle-sharing among addicts.

The spread of AIDS by needle exchange is not confined to adults. The Centers for Disease Control in Atlanta believes that among children under age 13, 40 percent of those with AIDS got the disease from their mother because she was shooting up and exchanging needles while pregnant or because the father's sperm carried the AIDS virus as a result of his drug abuse.

Still, allowing government agencies to hand out clean needles to addicts or giving tax money to private organizations to do the same thing has always seemed to me to be the equivalent of raising the white flag in the war on drugs.

When you live in a country where you can exchange your dirty needle for a clean one or a heroin addict can simply pick up a large supply of clean syringes at the drug store, aren't you living in a country that has given up on the drug problem?

Congress and our last two presidents certainly have seemed to think so. Since 1988, six federal laws have been passed containing provisions that expressly prohibit spending federal money on needle exchange programs. Many states also have laws that explicitly forbid the sale of needles and syringes without a medical prescription.

However, a report from the U.S. General Accounting Office contains some facts on the impact of needle exchange programs that make me think my concerns are misplaced.

The GAO examined all the published studies on needle exchange programs now running in Australia, Canada, the Netherlands, Sweden and the United Kingdom. The agency also took a close look at two small needle exchange programs that have been running for a couple of years in Tacoma, Wash., and New Haven, Conn.

The GAO found strong evidence that the rate of needle-sharing goes down as a result of the programs. Moreover, there is no evidence that the rate of drug addiction goes up as a result of the availability of clean needles.

Most impressive, and most surprising given my worries equating making needles available with writing off the addicts who use them, is the report's finding that needle exchange programs actually help addicts get into drug treatment programs as well as getting access to other health services, such as prenatal care for pregnant women.

The GAO took an especially close look at the needle exchange program in New Haven. The agency concluded that needle exchange has led to a 33 percent reduction in the number of new HIV infections associated with injecting drugs.

By gathering up old needles and getting clean ones out to addicts, the needle exchange program decreases the amount of time that infected needles are in use. Thus, the GAO report concludes that "such programs are effective."

It is hard to see how anyone can read this report and not come away thinking it is time for Congress to rethink its ban on allowing federal funds to be used to underwrite needle exchange.

It still do not much like the moral concession concerning drug use that is made when government gives needles to addicts. But a 33 percent reduction in HIV transmission, using a strategy that does not lead to an increase in drug use while actually helping get some addicts into treatment, is impressive enough for me to let reality intrude into my moral universe.

Maybe it is time for Congress, the president and state legislators to let a little reality into theirs.

Let's Make Sure TB Epidemic
Remains History

It's not their fault. The headline writers for the supermarket tabloids try as hard as they can to scare us. But, no matter how many would-be alien rapists or mummies-come-to-life leer at us while we buy our milk or onion dip, the scariest news and the most gut-twisting photographs are not found in the pages of the *Star*, the *Globe* or the *Enquirer*.

If you want something to really worry about, something you can sink your anxiety into, pick up any recent article in a medical or scientific journal on the subject of infectious diseases.

One of the most frightening photos I have ever seen appeared in *Science* magazine. The picture is of a tiny house in upstate New York. The boxy little place is freshly painted, has neatly pressed, white curtains in every window and a beautifully carved door. But this house is not what it appears to be. It was the first tuberculosis sanitarium built in the United States, and it made the magazine because there is reason to fear that it may be back in use soon.

At the turn of the century, more Americans died of tuberculosis than any other disease. Worldwide, tens of millions of people died from this dreaded bacteria—transmitted by contact with saliva or droplets from coughing or sneezing—that gets into and destroys the lungs.

Few are alive today who can remember the devastation that TB caused in this country. Improvements in sanitation, housing and diagnosis and the appearance during World War II of powerful drugs, such as penicillin, brought the disease to its knees. Probably only your grandparents or great-grandparents can remember the tales told by their parents about the plague that was TB.

Now, TB is back. The National Institutes of Health recently convened a meeting to discuss what to do about new strains of tuberculosis, which are immune to penicillin and other existing forms of antibiotics. Thirteen states, from New York to Hawaii, reported at least one case of drug-resistant TB in 1991. According to an article in *The New York Times*, New York City's Bellevue Hospital saw 62 patients with tuberculosis in one month, and 16 of them have TB that is not responding to drugs. These patients must be kept in isolation.

Admittedly, 16 patients is not a lot compared with the numbers of Americans struck down annually by heart disease, cancer, AIDS and accidents. But TB is highly contagious, and current tests do not reliably pick up the bacillus until it may be too late.

Ironically, those with AIDS are the primary victims of the new strains of deadly TB. Their weakened immune systems make them ripe for infection by bacteria, and the new virulent strains are attacking them first. There is, however, no reason to think that drug-resistant forms of TB will not spread to the general population.

The United States is poorly prepared to deal with TB. Doctors are no longer taught about the disease in medical school; there are almost no TB specialists in this country; and research funds for TB are minuscule.

Americans have seen what the AIDS virus did when the nation was slow to respond to it. A few scattered cases can quickly become an epidemic. We must not allow TB to become what AIDS has become. The time for action is now, so that the old sanitarium in upstate New York remains empty.

Thirty Years of Failure Followed
Surgeon General Tobacco Report

On Jan. 11, 1964, a physician from Red Level, Ala., Dr. Luther B. Terry, then the surgeon general of the United States, issued the most important public health document ever released by the federal government.

The report of the Surgeon General's Advisory Committee on Smoking and Health found, on the basis of more than 7,000 articles then published in scientific and medical journals, that cigarette smoking causes cancer and chronic bronchitis.

The report stated that "cigarette smoking is a health hazard of sufficient importance in the United States to warrant appropriate remedial action."

So how well has the federal government done in taking action with respect to smoking? The American Heart Association, American Lung Association and American Cancer Society issued a 30-year "report card" on the federal government's performance with respect to tobacco.

Looking over their grades, most federal agencies are going to be staying after school and putting in some hard time in the detention room.

One measure of our government's performance with respect to tobacco is the number of deaths caused by tobacco. By this standard, every administration since Lyndon Johnson's flunks. In 30 years, more than 2 million Americans have died from smoking-related lung cancer alone. Some 420,000 Americans died last year from tobacco-related diseases and illnesses.

Smokers are not the only victims of tobacco. Another 3,000 Americans die each year as a result of prolonged exposure to secondhand tobacco smoke. Twenty infants wind up hospitalized every day due to lung infections caused by secondhand tobacco smoke.

Are we really sure that tobacco smoking does all this damage?

Anyone inclined to doubt the conclusions of Terry's 1964 report can plow through the 23 subsequent surgeon generals' reports that reach the same conclusion or the roughly 60,000 scientific studies that link tobacco use with death and disease.

So the body count is clear and the cause is known. What has your government done about the problem? Well, according to the just-released report card, not much.

The White House gets an F from the lung, heart and cancer organizations. No president in 30 years has been willing to make tobacco control a policy priority.

The Federal Trade Commission also pulls an F. This agency, which has the authority to prevent unfair, misleading and deceptive advertising practices, has turned a blind eye to tobacco by allowing ads that promote smoking as a way to control weight, that falsely imply that low-tar and low-nicotine cigarettes are safe, and by not clamping down on ads that skirt the ban on advertising cigarettes on television and radio through the sponsorship of sports events.

The Food and Drug Administration scores an F for failing to take any steps to regulate tobacco products and for failing to try to expand its regulatory authority over tobacco products.

The Department of Agriculture also registers an F for its ongoing tobacco price support program that ensures farmers a minimum price for growing a deadly addictive substance.

The Office of the U.S. Trade Representative, which administers trade agreements with other countries, gets an F as well for trying hard for the past 30 years to promote the sale of American tobacco products in Third World countries.

Why can't our government get tough with tobacco? The answers are easy—money and a lack of drama.

The tobacco industry and the huge corporate conglomerates that own cigarette companies gave $9.3 million to congressional candidates over the last six years. Too many people are making too much money growing tobacco, peddling cigarettes, advertising them and representing tobacco's corporate interests in Washington.

The other reason for the lack of a tough government response is that tobacco kills slowly and insidiously. While new kids join the ranks of smokers every day, there are no dramatic photos or violent episodes surrounding smoking.

We are more afraid of teen-agers in gangs than we are of teen-agers who smoke and that is a big mistake. Because if we are ever going to put a real dent in the incredible harm caused by smoking, if we are ever to move toward affordable health care for all, we are going to have to get off our butts and make our public officials get tough on tobacco.

Columbus' Followers Brought
Diabetes to Indians, Too

Christopher Columbus is getting a lot of bad ink these days.

Back when I was a kid, in Paleolithic times, Columbus was the brave explorer who discovered the New World in order to assure all American children a day off from school. I recently visited a museum exhibit on Columbus and other early European explorers held to commemorate the 500th anniversary of the voyage of the Nina, the Pinta and the Santa Maria across the big pond. The trip was described as an "encounter." Christopher Columbus, "encounterer."

Columbus has truly become a 90's guy.

Many Americans resent the controversy surrounding the celebration of Columbus' voyage. But there is ample ground for controversy and debate over the quincentennial of his voyage.

Columbus was the edge of the wedge for European migration to the Americas. For the Indian peoples already here, the migration meant forced relocation, broken promises and war. Those times may seem long ago and far away. But Columbus set in motion a series of events that are still killing thousands of American Indians every year.

When Columbus arrived, he had few weapons and only a tiny number of soldiers. But he and his fellow Europeans had inadvertently brought along something that would prove far more deadly than weapons. They brought new foods and knowledge about how to produce them in abundance. These foods are still killing American Indians today.

One of every 1,000 members of the Tohono O'odham tribe, who live near Tucson, Ariz., dies of diabetes. In the last 20 years, the rate of diabetes among the members of the tribe has more than quadrupled. More than half of those over 40 have the disease.

The O'odham have, according to Richard Johnson in an eye-opening story in the June 21, 1992 *Denver Post*, the highest mortality rate from diabetes in the United States. They are 16 times more likely to develop diabetes than the average white American.

The staggeringly high rates of diabetes are not confined to the O'odham. About one-quarter of Colorado's Ute Indians over 45 have diabetes. The Pima Indians, who live near Phoenix, have the highest rate of diabetes in the world. More than half of all Pimas over the age of 35 are severely diabetic.

These astronomical rates of diabetes extract a terrible toll in terms of premature deaths, blindness and stroke. Severe diabetes causes impotency, threatening the very survival of these small tribes. Taxpayers spent nearly $70 million last year to provide dialysis, surgery and medicine to treat diabetic Native Americans.

What does Columbus have to do with the plague of diabetes ravaging Indians in the American Southwest? Many researchers think that Indians such as the O'odham, Utes and Pima have a unique biological ability to store fat.

Their ancestors, living at the time of Columbus' arrival, had to contend with a feast or famine environment of the desert. Tribes such as the O'odham seem to have evolved the ability to store fat so that they would have a source of calories in lean times.

But the genetic disposition to store fat has proven fatal as the legacy of Columbus reached Colorado and Arizona. Native foods such as prickly pear, carob and cholla cactus have been replaced by high-fat, high-sugar foods such as colas, cheeseburgers and beer. While these foods pose risks to the health of all Americans, they are especially dangerous for Native Americans whose genetic makeup predisposes them to obesity and early onset of diabetes.

The federal government spends less than 15 percent of its diabetes research budget on all minorities. Native Americans already cost the government five times that much every year in health care costs—and the bill is rising.

Columbus is not responsible for the fact that O'odham Indians can easily buy french fries. Native Americans who are genetically at high risk for diabetes need to learn to adjust their diets.

But those who followed him to these shores and brought their diet and culture with them need to do more to stop the epidemic of diabetes that is destroying the descendants of those who were already here when Columbus arrived. That would give both the critics and the admirers of Christopher Columbus something to celebrate.

Syphilis Study Increased Fear, Loathing

Syphilis is a major public-health problem in the United States.

The incidence of the disease, which is spread through sexual contact, has been exploding among young men. In 1982, the rate of infection was 14 per 100,000. By 1992, the rate had climbed to nearly 30 per 100,000. It's especially high among young black men.

Why don't more black men seek treatment? One reason is an experiment that took place in Alabama beginning more than 50 years ago.

Syphilis is an especially horrible disease. Once the bacteria enters the body, it can, over a period of years, cause paralysis, insanity and blindness. In 30 percent of untreated cases, syphilis leads to heart damage and death.

How do doctors know about the ravages of syphilis? Where do the medical journals and textbooks get their knowledge of this terrible disease? A key source of information is the Tuskegee study, one of the most morally heinous experiments ever conducted in the history of American health care.

From the 1940s to the early 1970s, the U.S. Public Health Service knowingly withheld penicillin, a reliable cure for syphilis, from 412 poor, illiterate black men in Macon County, Ala. The goal was to learn about the effects of syphilis by monitoring these men as the disease slowly ravaged their bodies and minds.

Not only was effective treatment withheld from these men, but they were never told they had syphilis. They were allowed to go home to their wives and lovers and spread the disease to others. No one knows exactly how many people died or were maimed as a result of the Tuskegee study.

The justification for the study was that since these men were illiterate and too poor to afford medical care, they would never get treatment for their disease. So those who ran the study—doctors; public-health officials and bureaucrats in Washington, D.C.; and doctors and nurses, black and white, in Alabama—convinced themselves that it was ethical to allow the men to go for decades without receiving a shot of penicillin.

And the knowledge has proven useful. During four decades, 14 papers were published in journals of medicine and public health about the effects of syphilis on the men in the study. What we know today about the decimating effects of syphilis on the heart, brain and joints is, in part, based on the Tuskegee study.

Five leading medical journals, including the *New England Journal of Medicine* and the *American Journal of Medicine*, have published articles that make explicit reference to the data derived from the Tuskegee study. None of these papers acknowledges the immoral circumstances under which the data were created.

The irony is that black men today still must contend with syphilis. Some because they do not have the money to afford medical care. Some because they are ignorant about the risks of unprotected sex. And some because they are afraid to go to the doctor as a result of what medicine did to poor black men in Macon County, Ala., decades ago.

Seek Safest, Cheapest, Best Cure
for World's Worst Child-Killer

Got any idea what is the biggest killer of children in the world today? It is not AIDS. Nor is it whooping cough or typhus. Accidents are not the culprit, either.

It is a medical problem that is almost never mentioned in polite company—diarrhea.

Sixty thousand kids die every day from this ailment. Five million babies and young children will die this year as a result of dehydration caused by diarrhea.

What you and I know about diarrhea is almost entirely a function of the tidal wave of commercials on TV and radio aimed at getting us to buy stuff at the drugstore to treat what the ads often tactfully call "indigestion" or "upset stomach." You know, the irritated tummy that everyone is troubled by at one time or another. The yukky problem that only a dancing cartoon stomach with a mouth or a giant fizzy tablet with a head can bring themselves to sing about by name.

In rich nations, diarrhea is a vaguely amusing, embarrassing disorder associated with eating and drinking too much. But, as David Werner makes clear in an important article in the journal *Pediatrics*, in poor countries diarrhea is no joke.

The inability of the nations of the world to figure out ways to get known treatments to the millions of kids who die is one of the great ethical failures of humankind.

Werner points out that for most of the world diarrhea is a problem that is the result of starvation, bad nutrition and poor sanitation. When children do not get enough to eat, their digestive systems go haywire and diarrhea is the result. The loss of water and important chemicals from the body causes the heart to fail and the kidneys to shut down. In too many places in the world a baby with diarrhea has a fatal illness.

There are, Werner says, two strategies for treating poor, starving kids with diarrhea. Both involve what is called rehydration therapy—getting water, salts and necessary chemicals back into the child as quickly as possible.

Fast rehydration can be accomplished by providing children and their families with what are called oral rehydration packets. These packets contain premixed amounts of glucose, salt, potassium and other chemicals that can quickly get the body's chemistry stable.

The other way to get the baby's body back in balance involves supplying the same chemicals in a form that can be added to the food or drink that families normally consume. Home mix can be prepared by a mom or dad and given to a child in traditional foods such as porridge, rice water, soup, gruel or drinks.

Both methods cure kids. Some experts, governments and international aid programs favor giving out premixed, self-contained packets. They believe that this is the safest and most reliable way to get the right mix of chemicals to a child in need because the packets leave no room for error or contamination.

Community health workers, such as Werner, argue that home mix is better because it is easier to keep on hand, easier to supply in nations with underdeveloped systems of communication and transportation, and makes the parents feel more involved in caring for their child.

There is another key difference between premixed packets and home mixes. Packets cost more. A family earning 50 cents a day may not have the 15 or 20 cents to spare to buy a premixed packet. Mixes cost only pennies.

Werner worries that the companies that are in the oral rehydration packet business have far more incentive to push packets than mixes.

The fact that, according to the World Health Organization, multinational drug companies last year sold $50 million worth of absolutely useless medications in poor countries for treating diarrhea in malnourished children lends support to the view that the bottom line may have more to do with the preference for packets rather than mixes.

The obvious solution to the epidemic of death caused by diarrhea in babies and young children is to solve the problem of malnutrition by making sure kids everywhere get enough to eat.

But until that goal is achieved, the nations of the world ought to rededicate themselves to making sure that no child dies of diarrhea by providing the safest, cheapest, most effective cure available—home rehydration mixes.

Individual Assignment: A Child's Health

In 1990, more than 10,000 American children younger than 5 got the measles. At least 60 of them died from complications of the disease. But in 1988, there were 3,400 cases of measles and only a handful of deaths.

Why the epidemic?

A lot of attention has focused on parents who refuse to get their kids immunized on religious or cultural grounds. But the measles epidemics ravaging Los Angeles, Philadelphia, Houston and Newark are not the result of religious. conviction conflicting with modern medicine. The problem is that America is indifferent to the health of its children.

In the United States, medical care for young children has deteriorated to the point at which newborns and toddlers have become susceptible to such preventable diseases as measles, rubella and whooping cough. In 1990, there were 11 babies born in the United States who were damaged by rubella; in 1988, there were two. Cases of whooping cough went from 2,823 in 1987 to 4,138 in 1990.

The state of the health of our children is a moral disgrace. According to D.A. Henderson, a professor of public health at Johns Hopkins University who led the World Health Organization's successful effort to eradicate smallpox, the United States has the third worst vaccination rate for children in the western hemisphere. Only Haiti and Bolivia vaccinate a smaller percentage of their kids.

Inadequate funding is one reason why our infant health care is on a par with that available in Belize and Paraguay. But money is not the only problem. Inadequate access to providers is the other major obstacle. In many inner-city neighborhoods and small rural towns, there are too few doctors, too few clinics and too many parents impaired by drugs, ignorance or alcohol to use the resources that do exist. Newborns in these situations need help. They need a health-care advocate.

In Minnesota, St. Paul's Department of Community Services has an innovative program to use public-health nurses and volunteers to go door-to-door to find pregnant women and give them phone numbers and information about health services. It is a great idea, but it does not go far enough.

In 1989, 4,021,000 children were born in the United States. There are 607,089 licensed physicians and more than 3 million licensed nurses in the country. It's time to bring them together. It should be a condition of licensure that every health-care professional be an advocate for the health care of one newborn baby for the first two years of that child's life.

In an "Advokids" program, each licensed doctor and nurse—and if the numbers are a little short, licensed dentist, pharmacist, social worker, hospital administrator and psychologist—would be assigned a child born in the state where the health-care practitioner is licensed. To stay licensed, the professional would have to certify that he or she has contacted the mother of that child within one week after birth to see if any problems have arisen and to make sure there is postnatal care for baby and mom. Those in the Advokids program would have to remain in contact with their assigned children for the next two years, making sure the kids get their shots and that the parents know how to get health care if a problem arises.

No one, including doctors, nurses and other health-care professionals, likes to be told to do something for nothing. But the problem for young kids in our health-care system is that we treat them as if they are nothing. It is time to make sure that every child has at least one health-care provider who treats him or her as somebody.

U.S. Needs Preventive Medicine for
Its Epidemic of Violence

Concern about violent crime is never far from the minds of most Americans. A report by the National Academy of Sciences, "Understanding and Preventing Violence," shows why.

This landmark report—whose authors include a distinguished group of sociologists, criminologists, psychologists and biologists—has a lot to say about how bad the problem is, who is responsible, and what we should and should not do about violent crime.

The United States is, the report observes, the most violent industrialized nation in the world. Our murder rates far exceed those in other comparable countries. This country has the highest rates for sexual and all other forms of personal assault. One-third of the 19 million crimes that were reported in 1990 involved violence.

Violence is a major threat to the health of all Americans. It may come as a small comfort that you are living in what is only the third most violent era of this century in America.

The most violent period of the 20th century in this country occurred in the early 1930s. Murders and other violent acts then decreased until they suddenly shot up between 1979 and 1981. We temporarily cut back on the number of rapes, murders, assaults and robberies committed against one another only to return to the repellent rates of 1980 in recent years.

Minorities are at the greatest risk of suffering from violence. The National Academy study states that blacks are 41 percent more likely and Hispanics 32 percent more likely to be the victims of violent crime than are whites. A young black man is 20 times more likely to suffer violent crime than an older white female.

Death and injury are not the only price to be paid for the plague of violence that the report finds plagues this nation. It costs $54,000 to cope with the consequences of a rape attempt, $19,200 per robbery, $16,000 per assault.

In addition to paying these huge sums for lost productivity, medical costs, psychological damage and law enforcement, each of us pays an almost unimaginable toll in terms of the damage done to our neighborhoods, the deterioration of our cities and the psychic toll on our quality of life.

So who is responsible? The report points the finger of blame straight at young men who are disproportionately members of minority groups. Those who commit acts of violence are usually acquaintances of their victims in a majority of assaults, rapes and homicides.

The report debunks the idea that violent crime is the work of violent career criminals. Only a few individuals commit violent crimes frequently. Most violent crime is committed by offenders who have some non-violent criminal violations on their record, but no previous history of violent crime.

Perhaps the single most important finding in the report is that our current approach to battling violent crime—incarceration—is a dismal failure. The average prison time served for violent crime tripled between 1975 and 1989 without making so much as a dent in the number of violent crimes.

While politicians find it easy to blather on about stiffer sentences and tougher penalties, the blunt truth is that "a further increase in the average time served per violent crime would have an even smaller ... effect" than did tripling the average prison term over the past 15 years.

Prison is expensive and it does not work. We need more innovative solutions to the crisis of violence. The report suggests that prevention rather than deterrence is the direction in which we need to head.

It calls for programs that can prevent aggression and violence among children, the redesign of buildings and workplaces to lessen the chance of violence, interventions to prevent alcohol and drug abuse, and counseling programs and public education campaigns to reduce partner and sexual assaults.

Perhaps the most controversial suggestions are that studies be launched to identify medications that can reduce violent behavior and to find signs that indicate which individuals are at greatest risk for committing violent acts.

There is a grave danger that studies of the biology of violence or research to find drugs to reduce the disposition toward violence might become ways to avoid grappling with the poverty and poor social conditions that breed crime. And one cannot go far down the path of biology without encountering the pit of racism.

Still, the report seems to be on track when it says that it is time to admit that our existing responses to violent crime have failed and we had better set about finding different strategies emphasizing prevention rather than punishment.

It is not that we should coddle violent criminals or excuse what they do. It is simply that whatever the form of punishment we administer, it is always too late for the victim and does little to make the rest of us feel more secure about ourselves and our families. We need to spend less time figuring out how to punish violent criminals and more time figuring out how to prevent their behavior.

U.S. at Last Has Rejoined Rest of World
in Recognizing Population Problem

Last Thursday I spent the morning getting depressed by former Colorado Sen. Timothy Wirth.

Wirth was depressing me because that is part of his job. President Clinton appointed him undersecretary of state for global affairs. In that capacity, it is Wirth's sworn duty to scare the bejeebers out of you and me about the fact that there are way too many people living on the Earth.

Wirth is good at his job. He appeared at the University of Minnesota's Humphrey Institute at the first of four town meetings around the country on World Population and Sustainable Development.

As I tried to figure out if I was awake enough to get my coffee cup up anywhere near my mouth, Wirth looked directly at me and asked if I was aware that there were currently 5.7 billion of us hanging around the planet.

I confessed I was not, although I added lamely that the traffic I had battled coming to the university meant that a lot of those people had cars and were not afraid to drive them in 10 below zero weather.

Wirth managed a polite smile. Then he raised an issue that really got my attention. Did I know that, presuming no change in our collective reproductive habits, there will be twice that number trying to squeeze onto the globe by the year 2030? Nearly all of the increase in numbers will take place in the poorest nations of the world.

If the predicted increase in numbers happens, he warned, the growth in the number of mouths to feed will swamp any effort any government can make to protect the environment, maintain biodiversity, save wetlands, preserve forests, provide economic opportunity to the young or guarantee a minimum of education and health care for all.

If all that wasn't depressing enough, Wirth said that, of the roughly 6 billion people expected to be here around the year 2000, about 2 billion of them will be teenagers. Given teen-age romantic proclivities, there is a lot of work ahead of us all if the explosion in the world's population is to be in any way reduced.

Wirth came to Minnesota to talk about the plans that the Clinton administration has for dealing with the population crisis at the World Population Conference to be held in September, 1994 in Cairo, Egypt. This is the third in a series of once-every-decade conferences sponsored by the United Nations to talk about population issues.

John Sharpless, a professor of history at the University of Wisconsin and an expert on the history of modern efforts to rein in population growth, noted that Wirth and the Clinton administration are finally moving to take on the population issue after a decade of neglect by Presidents Bush and Reagan.

In the 1980s the question of doing something about the population crisis was linked to the issue of elective abortion. Family planners here and in other nations argued that access to safe abortion had to be a part of the overall strategy for providing women with options to control their own fertility.

But talk of abortion made the population issue taboo for Reagan and Bush. Wirth's predecessor, James Buckley, was sent by Reagan to the last U.N. conference in 1984 in Mexico City.

There, in one of the most overpopulated, sickeningly polluted and befouled cities in the world, Buckley declared that there was no world population crisis. He declaimed that the only crisis was economic as a result of the insufficient embrace of free market capitalism by underdeveloped nations.

The current administration has given up on this fantasy. Wirth and the other delegations from around the world who will be in Cairo in September all seem to agree that there are too many people in too many places on the earth. The question is what to do to solve the problem.

When our folks show up in Cairo they will argue that the key to getting a handle on population is to make sure that women who want family planning services, including access to safe methods of abortion, have them. Empowering women will lead to fewer children.

They will also argue that another key to reducing population is to convince men and women that they need not have lots of children either to insure that some will live to adulthood or to insure their own security as they age. Better health care and more economic development will take away the incentive that exists in many parts of the world to have lots of children.

But to be effective moral leaders we must not be seen as hypocritical. And that is one of the problems America faces as the Cairo meeting approaches. The United States currently has no population policy of its own. It will be hard to tell other nations that they ought to have policies when we do not.

We are spending lots of money on medical procedures aimed at enhancing and extending fertility. It will be hard to tell those in other nations that they should have fewer children if we are doing everything we can to help women in their late 50s have them.

And we are not going to seem especially credible to the rest of the world about our commitment to their health if we spend $2 million in a long-shot effort to save a Siamese twin while not spending the pennies it would take to easily prevent the hundreds of thousands of deaths that take place each year around the world from polio, diarrhea, hepatitis and malnutrition.

The current administration has joined the rest of the world in recognizing that there is a population problem. There is no consensus on what to do about that problem. The only way we can hope to influence the solution is to do what we can to minimize the gap between our moral rhetoric and our actions.

China's Proposal to Discourage "Inferior" Births Unjust, Immoral

One of the biggest stories of the year got barely any media attention.

Bill Clinton's alleged dalliances under the vigilant eyes of the Arkansas state police got many column inches. Michael Jackson's nocturnal practices took up hours of radio and television time.

But, the stated intention of the leaders of the world's most heavily populated nation to pursue a vigorous national policy of eugenics was barely a blip on the media radar screen.

In mid-December, 1993 the Chinese government made public a bill entitled "On Eugenics and Health Protection." The aim of the proposed law is very clear. China's legislators believe that the more than ten million Chinese born each year with birth defects and disabilities "could have been prevented through better controls." The easiest, cheapest and most effective way to deal with the "problem" is to prevent births of "inferior quality."

The prevention strategies the Chinese have in mind would bring a blush to the cheek of some of the self-appointed generals in America's rearguard war against sexuality: Pat Robertson, Andrea Dworkin, Catherine Mackinnon and Cal Thomas.

One method is to "urge" those at risk of giving birth to children with problems, such as mothers who have hepatitis, to seek the permission of the state prior to procreation. Another is to "encourage" mothers found to be carrying children with birth defects such as spina bifida, deafness, mental retardation or AIDS to terminate their pregnancies.

Still another is to simply sterilize those who have a history of retardation or mental illness.

Since China has been diligently enforcing a one child per family rule for many years, including coerced abortions when necessary, no one should doubt the present government's ability to put eugenic theory into practice.

The announcement by the Chinese that they intend to improve the health of their nation by eliminating the unfit and the disabled was greeted with almost no comment by Western governments. The decision to go eugenic as a matter of Chinese national policy was treated as if the largest nation on earth had emitted a large belch in otherwise polite company.

American specialists in foreign affairs and the pundits who love them apparently find the threat of a North Korean atomic bomb in the hands of a goofball leftover regime from the Cold War more frightening than the Chinese policy. Not only has our government remained mum about the Chinese plan to institute a coercive national policy of eugenics, some of the diplomatic denizens of Foggy Bottom have recently been burbling in glowing terms about the improved human rights climate in the nation where a quarter of the world's people live.

J. Stapleton Roy, our ambassador to China, is quoted in the *New York Times* as being of the opinion that over the past 150 years of Chinese history, "the last two years are the best in terms of prosperity, individual choice ... and stable domestic conditions." Well, life may well be better for the average Chinese citizen than at any time since the Opium Wars, and things may be a lot more stable than they were when —during the heady days of the Cultural Revolution under the watchful eye of Mao—the Red Guard was rousting the ideologically deviant out of their beds for a mandatory trip to a labor camp.

But contrary to the ambassador's opinion, individual choice is not doing well and will take a precipitous nosedive on the diplomatic human rights scoreboard if the authorities implement a policy of policing the bedroom and the obstetrics ward with an eye toward improving the species.

The Chinese eugenics policy deserves a much, much more vigorous response than American and other world leaders have mustered to date. Undoubtedly this has little to do with the desire of the United States and Europe to increase trade.

But, the Clinton administration should make it clear that there will be no progress on trade unless coercive eugenics is no longer a part of Chinese reproductive policy. When a nation says that it will do everything in its power to coerce, bully and threaten its citizens into getting rid of the deviant, the disordered and the disabled, the international community must speak out.

Such a patently immoral course of action is no more tolerable today than it was 50 years ago when, inspired by the loopy dreams of German race hygienists, the Nazis were polishing off the infirm, the insane and the supposedly inferior in Dachau, Beltzen, Buchenwald and Auschwitz.

CHAPTER 7
GENETICS

Genetic Registry to Be
Filled with Data, Dilemmas

If you are a thorough newspaper reader, you may be one of the few people to know that your government is about to take a giant leap forward in the march to apply genetic knowledge to your life.

If you read your newspaper very, very carefully, you might have seen a squib of a story buried on a back page about the Defense Depart-ment announcing plans to create a huge registry of genetic information.

Why, when even the most modest experiment with human genes generates an ethics maelstrom, did one of the most important developments in the history of applied genetics—the creation of the world's first large-scale, government-sponsored genetic registry—fail to dent the nation's collective awareness?

The goal of the Defense Department in creating a DNA repository is very simple. The armed services want to create an enormous file of genetic "fingerprints" that could be used to help identify bodily remains. Every soldier in the armed services would be required to provide some cells obtained by either drawing a tiny bit of blood from a finger or a swab of the mouth. The sample will be kept on a card in a huge refrigerated vault.

If someone should be killed in an airplane crash or on the battlefield where only a few incomplete bodily remains are found, DNA could still be extracted from these remains and then matched against the DNA extracted from some of the cells on the sample kept in the national registry. By using new techniques to match patterns between samples of DNA, very precise identification would be possible.

Now, there is absolutely nothing unethical about trying to come up with a more reliable method of identifying who it is that has died in an accident or a war. Unknown soldier casualties are especially tragic for families and friends left wondering about their loved ones. But there are important ethical and policy questions that should be asked about any effort to create genetic registries.

Who will have access to the information stored in the armed services DNA repository? Could a district attorney subpoena the samples for testing in criminal proceedings? What if a serviceman were involved in alleged theft in a conservative Moslem nation, where the penalty for robbery is the amputation of an arm or death? Would the Defense Department honor a request for DNA identification of hair or blood found at the scene of the crime?

Will the Defense Department honor requests to crosslink its DNA files with those of military police agencies? What about with civilian police departments or the FBI? Can researchers study the files for any purpose they want?

And, what about requests from insurance companies or employers to check the files once new tests for detecting dispositions to disease by analyzing DNA come on-line in the next few years? Would the military itself be able to resist the temptation to scour its own DNA files to see who might develop mental illness, cancer, diabetes, heart disease or any of a number of other potentially expensive disabilities and ailments? And what if a mistake were made in the collection and storage of samples? Is there any provision for a person to ask for a recheck of his sample in the DNA bank?

Collecting large amounts of biological material for DNA testing will bring many benefits to the armed services and, ultimately, to society. But there are a number of hard questions that need to be answered about the rules and principles that should govern these registries. The time to start answering them is now.

Genetic Snoops Should Leave
Lincoln Alone

Remember the television commercial in which Abraham Lincoln, who's looking for an executive position, is humiliated by a job counselor?

"You got no college education, no sheepskin buddy," the counselor sniffs. "We'll get back to you." A chastened Lincoln shuffles off knowing a leadership position is not in the cards.

Well, Honest Abe is about to go through a different sort of wringer. One hundred twenty-five years after his death, scientists want to see if he had the biological stuff of which leaders are made.

The National Museum of Health and Medicine in Washington, D.C., appointed a committee of doctors and scientists to decide whether samples of Lincoln's hair, bone and blood—kept at the museum since his autopsy—should be subjected to genetic analysis.

The researchers want to know if Lincoln had a genetic condition known as Marfan's syndrome. Marfan's causes those who have it to grow tall and gangly. It also causes abnormalities in the bones, joints and blood vessels. About 40,000 Americans have this genetic disease.

The scientists are thinking about taking a tiny sample of Lincoln's tissue, extracting his DNA from the cells, and copying it thousands of times to get enough genetic material to run the newly available test for Marfan's.

Neat technology, but a bad idea. A retrospective autopsy of the genes of an historic figure like Lincoln for no pressing reason smacks more of voyeurism than of science. What if the genetic sleuths discover that Lincoln's DNA contains some other genetic anomaly—say Huntington's disease, or an abnormal extra chromosome?

Would Lincoln want such things known? Do researchers, you or I have the right to know them simply because Lincoln is not here to invoke his right to privacy?

If scientists are encouraged to satisfy our curiosity about Lincoln's biology, who will be next? Will *People* magazine start a new "bad seed" feature? Will "Inside Edition" reveal that Al Capone really did suffer from XYY syndrome? Will other presidents, their families or other public figures need to embargo their mortal remains to prevent unwanted genetic snooping by subsequent generations?

There is no fun in arguing that there are facts out there that ought not be known—especially when it would be easy to get the facts, and when those who might be hurt by their disclosure are long since dead.

There is no reason to suppose that Lincoln would object to what the scientists want to do. But doesn't it make more sense to encourage efforts to understand and appreciate Lincoln's legacy through his words and deeds rather than through his DNA?

To Be Safe, Screen Risks,
Not Workers

On Oct. 10, 1990, the U.S. Supreme Court heard arguments in the Johnson Controls case. Johnson Controls is a Milwaukee-based company that manufactures automobile batteries. Because some of the chemicals used in making the batteries may cause birth defects in a developing fetus, the company instituted a policy barring any woman capable of bearing a child from the factory floor. Some women at Johnson Controls are fighting the policy on the grounds that the company is practicing gender selection.

At first glance, the case looks like a classic confrontation between the rights of women to work and the rights of fetuses to be born healthy. In his argument before the Supreme Court, one of the lawyers for Johnson Controls framed the issues involved in just that way. He argued that Congress, in passing laws against sex discrimination in employment, did not mean to "require an employer to damage unborn children."

The lawyer is right about congressional intent, but his defense of the Johnson Controls policy misses what is at stake here. The issue is not whether fetal rights or women's rights are more deserving of legal protection. It's whether employers should be allowed to deal with hazards in the workplace by excluding workers on the basis of their biology.

A report, "Genetic Monitoring and Screening in the Workplace," issued by the Office of Technology Assessment, makes it clear that the Supreme Court decision in the Johnson Controls case will have implications for all Americans—men and women. The report analyzes genetic tests soon to become available that will reveal who among us is most likely to get diabetes, cancer, hypertension, severe depression or multiple sclerosis. In order to control their skyrocketing health costs, companies will be eager to avoid hiring those who these tests predict are most likely to get sick.

Genetic-screening tests also will be widely available soon. These tests can detect genetic damage in a tiny blood sample, allowing accurate predictions as to which men and women are in danger of contracting costly illness as a result of exposure to substances in the workplace.

There are no laws protecting workers—men or women—from compulsory genetic monitoring in the workplace. Nor are there any laws prohibiting employers from requiring genetic screening as a precondition of employment.

The exclusion of women from the workplace is actually a crude form of genetic screening. If the Supreme Court lets Johnson Controls exclude fertile women from the workplace today, if the company is allowed to say that all those who do not have a Y chromosome must go, companies will have a green light to begin using genetic screening to exclude you from your job or health or life insurance tomorrow.

The obvious solution to resolving the apparent clash of interests between women and fetuses is to make the workplace safe. Businesses should be required to create work environments that do not harm fetuses. Risks should be minimized by changing the workplace—not by excluding particular workers.

Allowing today's employers to solve workplace dangers by detecting and booting out those who face special risks means that, in the future, jobs will go not to those who can do the best work but to those who possess the best genes.

Ignorance About Genetic Testing
Raises Perils for Society

Do you know what genetic testing is? How about gene therapy? If you don't, you are not alone.

According to a telephone survey of 1,000 Americans conducted for the March of Dimes Birth Defects foundation, 68 percent of those polled said they knew relatively little or almost nothing about genetic testing and 86 percent said the same about gene therapy.

This dismal news arrives at a time when the federal government plans to spend $3 billion of your tax money over the next 15 years on a massive study, the human genome project, to crack the code of human heredity. That is about the amount of time we have to overcome our ignorance in order to prepare to deal with the enormous public policy challenges this information will create.

Ignorance about genetics is easy to understand. It takes no skill to manage to get all the way through high school and even college in the United States without ever taking a course in biology, much less genetics.

Even those few souls who do wind up taking a high school biology course are all too likely to take one that goes easy on the details of genetics often to placate those who adhere to biblical creationist accounts of how you and I came to be on this planet.

The result is that the average American has no idea what a gene is or how heredity actually works over time in our species. The March of Dimes survey gives plenty of reason for concern about the price of ignorance.

It found that 80 percent of Americans say they would take a genetic test before having a child if the test might indicate that the child would inherit a fatal genetic disease. Two out of three say they would take a test during pregnancy to determine whether the fetus had any genetic disease. The proportion of those who say they want genetic tests is even higher in those of childbearing age.

What is scary about these numbers is that people want testing even though most of us have little idea of what a hereditary disease is, what the chances are of passing it on or the fact that genetic diseases often show very different levels of severity from person to person.

If we do not do something to educate ourselves about the rapidly evolving science of genetics, it will not be long before doctors, lawyers and public officials are preying on our ignorance and anxieties to make sure that "responsible" parents undergo every possible form of genetic testing.

There are still more eye-catching findings in the survey. Fifty-eight percent of those polled said their insurance company should be informed of the results of genetic tests. And one-third said the person's employer should get test results.

It is hard to imagine the same results if drug or psychological testing were substituted for genetic testing. Yet, genetic tests are even more likely to reveal intimate and personal facts of the sort that few people would really want to involuntarily share with their insurance agent or boss.

The spookiest finding of the survey is that 43 percent of those responding said they approve of using genetic engineering or gene therapy to improve children's physical characteristics or intelligence. Well over one-third of Americans apparently see no problem with the idea that we ought to use knowledge about human genetics to try to design the perfect baby.

Recent 20th century history with its race-hygiene-motivated euthanasia programs and "ethnic cleansings" ought to leave us all rather humble in the face of talk about eugenics.

Before we decide to engineer out all the frailties, foibles and flaws in our species, it might be a good idea to sit down and think about what traits and characteristics really are "better" or "perfect" and why.

A society that knows as little about genetics, genetic testing and gene therapy as the March of Dimes survey indicates ought to proceed with extreme caution before trying to apply that knowledge to the next generation.

Radio Ranting Missed Point
of Birth Rights

In late November, 1991, the Federal Communications Commission, which grants licenses to radio and television stations, received a very unusual complaint.

A group of disability-rights activists claimed that on a radio program broadcast July 22, 1991 by KFI radio in Los Angeles, talk-show host Jane Norris unfairly, maliciously and repeatedly slurred people with disabilities.

Did Norris commit the unpardonable sin of deviating from the politically correct line? Or is there substance to the complaint?

Specifically, Norris spent most of her time on the air that day hyperventilating as to whether Bree Walker Lampley, a television news anchor at KCBS-TV in Los Angeles, was doing the right thing in having a baby with her husband and co-anchor, Jim Lampley (formerly seen on ABC college football telecasts).

Norris felt entitled to pose her ditsy question because the Lampleys knew that there was a 50/50 chance any baby they had would have the same disability—electrodactylism—that the mother has. Electrodactylism is a hereditary condition in which the bones of the hands and feet fuse together. If you have the condition, you probably can open a door but you won't play the piano.

Last week, I listened to a tape of Norris' show. Even by the let-it-all-hang-out standards some stations are encouraging their talk-jocks to use in an effort to preserve the dinosaur of AM radio, Norris' little stroll down eugenics lane was an unseemly display.

She kept wailing away at the idea that any kid born with fused fingers and toes would inevitably live a life of hell. "Is it fair," she incessantly asked, "to have a child that you know has a very good chance of contracting this deformity?"

The fact that Bree Walker Lampley has managed to live a life of fame and accomplishment while pulling in what must be some pretty big bucks as a prominent media personality didn't prevent Norris from repeatedly asking this question for nearly an hour. Nor did the fact that the Lampleys already have a child with the condition. The most unfair aspect of what is a notably low moment in public discourse is that no one with any disability experience is given a chance to point out that life can still be enjoyed even with dysfunctional fingers and toes.

Still, I would not penalize KFI or Norris for the boorish interlude. Norris was only doing what lots of folks do in the media these days—plumb the depths of controversy in an inflammatory manner to attract an audience. Mewing about the decision of local celebrities to have a baby who might have a genetic defect is little different from the subjects that leave Phil, Oprah and Sally in phony moral outrage.

If the FCC is going to yank the licenses of those who pander on the airwaves, a strange and eerie silence will descend upon the land. The real lesson to be learned from the discussion of the reproductive rights of Bree and Jim Lampley is that our society is moving full-steam ahead toward a confrontation with the social implications of advances in genetics. In a few years, it will be possible to detect such common hereditary conditions as cystic fibrosis, juvenile diabetes and polycystic kidney disease.

Those in the disability movement—and all the rest of us—need to be sure that no one seriously suggests making reproductive rights contingent on having the "right" genes.

Let's Listen to Arguments
About Deafness

Would you choose to have a child who is deaf? Before you answer, let me try to explain why that question soon will move from the realm of hypothesis to that of ethical dilemma.

Many older women and women who have previously had a child with a birth defect undergo amniocentesis when they are pregnant. During this procedure, tiny amounts of fluid are removed from the sac that protects the fetus. By analyzing cells in the fluid, doctors who are expert in the science of genetics can tell whether the fetus has certain genetic defects.

Amniocentesis and other prenatal tests available today can identify only a limited number of genetic problems. But that is about to change. Now under way at many universities is a federally sponsored human-genome project. The goal of the research is to map and sequence each of our genes, the bits of DNA that control heredity. The project began in 1990, and it is expected to last about 15 years.

The genome project will supply medical science with a complete, high-resolution genetic blueprint. When it does, all sorts of information will be available about who is at risk for getting cancer, heart disease, schizophrenia, Alzheimer's, muscular dystrophy and a host of other unpleasant maladies. The problem that doctors, nurses and counselors will face is how to explain all the risks and probabilities without scaring you to death.

Nowhere will the range of choices offered by genetic knowledge be more controversial than in the domain of reproduction. And this brings me back to my question about the deaf child. Some forms of deafness are hereditary. When couples who are deaf have children, they face a very high probability that any child they have will be deaf, too.

You may be thinking it must be tough to face those odds. But for some disorders, the human-genome project will allow doctors to tell precisely which embryos or fetuses carry the genetic message that produces hereditary deafness. When we learn the specific code for deafness, medicine will be able to prevent this form of the condition by allowing parents to identify and abort embryos or fetuses with the defective code.

But as a distinguished physician who has studied hereditary deafness for many decades wondered during a recent talk, exactly which fetus or embryo will deaf parents choose to abort? Many people who are deaf have grown up in families where parents and grandparents are also deaf. They may have brothers and sisters who are deaf. They may have gone to school with others who are deaf. They may speak only American Sign Language in their home, on the job and at family reunions. They have acculturated to their deafness.

For those who have adapted to it, deafness is not a defect. Many of those who are deaf do not see themselves as disabled. In fact, some deaf parents are so at ease with deafness that they hope their children will be deaf, too.

That's right. If given the choice, some people who are deaf and proud of who they are and secure in what they can do would voluntarily choose to have a deaf child. The genome project will allow them their choice. It is possible that while many couples might want to prevent the birth of a child who is deaf, there are some who would abort a fetus that would have had normal hearing in favor of one who would be deaf.

The results of the genome project will soon be upon us. We had better start communicating with each other, whether by word or sign, if we are going to deal with that knowledge wisely.

Being Petite is No Disease:
Why Try to Cure It?

If you are short, this is your time in the limelight. Every four years a passel of short people become our national heroes as they prance, tumble and leap across our television screens in the Olympics.

If you are much over 5 feet 4 you can forget about winning a gold on the balance beam or in floor exercise. Tall folks need not apply.

Matters are different on all other days for those who are short. Hey, shrimp! How's it going short stuff? How are ya doin', runt? These unhappy phrases and other even less felicitous ones are all too familiar to every American kid who is short.

I know because when I was a kid I rarely missed a chance to issue one of these zingers myself. And it is not just my presumedly mature and now more delicate sensibilities which are offended by ragging of this sort.

Study after study shows that, other things being equal, our society favors tall people over short ones for positions of leadership, authority, high incomes and power.

Suppose you and your spouse were very short. What if you found out that there was a new treatment, a hormone, that could alter your children's chemistry so that they would be taller than you. Would you want your child's height "treated?"

Lots of parents are saying "yes." For the question is no longer hypothetical. Parents all around America are pestering their doctors to use a new synthetic hormone on their kids so that they will not be short. Many pediatricians are giving human growth hormone to kids who lag behind on the normal growth curve, even though the side-effects of long-term administration of the hormone are not known.

For many years the National Institutes of Health, with the support of Eli Lilly, the pharmaceutical giant, has been conducting a study to see what effect synthetic growth hormone has on children's height.

Eighty healthy kids, ranging in age from 9-15, are in the study. There is nothing wrong with them except that their growth rates indicate that the girls will not be any taller than 4 feet 11 inches and the boys 5 feet 4 inches. Half the kids in the study are getting shots of human growth hormone three times a week. The other half only get placebo shots.

Recent breakthroughs in biotechnology are behind this effort to do something about short stature. For decades the only source of human growth hormone was pituitary glands taken from the brains of dead bodies. Growth hormone was in such short supply that the small amount available was given to children diagnosed as suffering from extreme dwarfism.

But, thanks to biotechnology, it is now possible to make human growth hormone in the lab. Eli Lilly and Genentech hold the patents on the synthetic hormone. At $10,000 or more for a year's supply, they stand to make a lot of money if every short kid in North America gets three injections of the stuff a week for 10 years.

Jeremy Rifkin, a well-known critic of biotechnology, threatened to sue the National Institute for Child Health and Human Development to shut down the federal study. Rifkin and his allies argue that the government is sponsoring a study to find a medical solution to what is a non-medical problem. I think he has a point.

The problem is not, as Rifkin and other critics of biotechnology allege, the application of genetic knowledge to solve medical problems. What could possibly be wrong with trying to cure genetic diseases such as sickle cell disease, hemophilia or Fanconi's anemia?

The ethical problem is that being short, in and of itself, is not a disease. If someone is unusually, atypically short because they do not produce growth hormone, it is reasonable to try and replace that deficiency.

But, is a boy or girl whose chemistry is normal but who still will grow up to be on the short side really to be thought of as "sick," "diseased" or "deformed"? Does a cultural prejudice against short people mean that doctors ought to tell kids destined to be short that they need medical treatment?

It is unethical for medicine and pharmaceutical companies to prey on yet another form of human insecurity to make a buck.

And, it is morally bananas for doctors to spend their time and energy figuring out what to do with kids who are somewhat shorter than average when there are so many other obvious, clearcut medical problems and disorders that continue to ravage children in this and other countries.

The kids in the ongoing federal study should be told that they will grow up shorter than average but that perhaps they will be able to compete as Olympic gymnasts or divers.

The pediatricians should put away their syringes and go after some real diseases. The cure for short stature is for the rest of us to grow up about it.

Don't Let "Jurassic Park" Terrify
Us About Genetic Engineering

It is *hideous*! It is *monstrous*! It is *incredible*! It is *targeted at your children*! *No one can stop it*!

That's right, "Jurassic Park" is finally at your local video store.

When Hollywood and science mix, watch out. Those who make movies like their scientists mad, bad and more than a tad morally zonkers. From Dr. Frankenstein and his goofing around with corpses and electricity to the folks in white coats whose nuclear shenanigans brought you Godzilla and Mothra, the silver screen has had few kind words for nerds with advanced degrees in science and technology.

"Jurassic Park" falls smack in the cinematic tradition that holds that science ain't no friend of yours or mine. Forget about the fact that the movie itself, loaded as it is with special effects and 20-foot-tall robots, is a pure paean to technology. The driving message of the book and the movie is that the price of progress in science and technology is too high in terms of the cost to human dignity and morality.

Many within the scientific community are simply battening down the hatches until the hype blows over. They figure a single summer blockbuster is not going to have the townsfolk organizing themselves into a vigilante party to set fire to the local gene therapy institute. Others are not so sure.

A couple of biologist friends have confided to me that they are already tired of explaining at every picnic, barbecue or cocktail party why they would not be tempted, even if they knew how, to try to recreate a dinosaur from an ancient DNA sample. They say they are not sure what to say when a backyard philosopher asks if they think it is OK to fool with Mother Nature's secrets when everything from their dog to their salad represents the results of mankind's manipulating nature.

I think those in the scientific community who argue for either ignoring or simply blowing off the "Jurassic Park" phenomena is just so much Mad Scientist nonsense are missing a great opportunity. While the themes of science out of control and a science indifferent to human values do not accurately describe what is taking place in genetics today, "Jurassic Park" does accurately reflect a set of anxieties about genetic engineering that have deep roots in our culture.

People are worried about what the "experts" are up to with respect to genetic engineering. They are concerned that they are going to find some unhealthy adulterated product on their grocery shelf that represents a large company's best effort to make a buck by genetically engineering milk, fruit or meat. They worry when they learn that researchers have already bred a goat-sheep hybrid, a "geep" in the jargon of genetics, without seeming to have needed permission or authorization from any agency or review board.

Genetic engineering does require more debate and discussion than it has received to date. But our key institutions are not well positioned to instigate that discussion. Most legislators and public officials cannot tell a chromosome from a chrome bumper. Our churches and schools are not adequately preparing the next generation for the choices they will face about how to use our rapidly expanding knowledge of heredity. And those who work in the media and the arts are frighteningly ignorant about genetics and biology.

The proof of our ignorance is right up there on the screen. We and our kids are not really sure what these gene jockeys are up to in their laboratories. We have no idea what sorts of regulations or rules govern their research, what motives or visions inspire their work.

Perhaps most frustrating is the fact that it is fear rather than hope that dominates "Jurassic Park." For while there are reasons for concern about where we are headed with genetic engineering and gene therapy, there are more reasons for excitement. As science slowly unravels the mysteries of heredity, medicine, agriculture and veterinary science will change for the better.

Molecular engineering will allow us to prevent diseases such as cystic fibrosis, sickle cell anemia and muscular dystrophy. We will be able to create animals that don't require massive amounts of antibiotics to fend off diseases. And we should be able to engineer plants that can grow in hot, arid climates—making famine nothing more than a horrid memory.

When you and your kids are talking about "Jurassic Park" and they are full of questions about dinosaurs and mad scientists, tell them there are reasons for concern about how well humanity will handle the secrets of heredity. But warn them too that they need to be concerned that our fear of genetic engineering not blind us to its potential enormous benefits.

Job Worries Distorting Concerns About Health Effects of BST

The other morning I awoke, stumbled down the stairs, staggered over to the cupboard and—to the grimacing dismay of my family—hauled out a box of Lucky Count Chokula Fortified Flakes so as to ingest my requisite morning dose of sugar and food coloring.

My wife attempted to shield my 9-year-old son's eyes from the dietary disaster. An accusatory "How can you eat that stuff?" rang out like a shot. I was too comatose to respond.

I trudged toward the fridge to grab some milk. We only keep skim in the house so this dimension of breakfast stirs no controversy. But I found myself wondering, what is going to happen in the Caplan household when milk obtained from cows that have been given bovine somatotropin (BST) starts appearing in the dairy case at the supermarket? If I insist on mixing milk from cows revved up on BST with my marshmallow-flavored Sunlight Crunchberries, will I wind up dining alone in the basement?

After more than a decade of controversy, the Food and Drug Administration has given its approval for the use of the genetically engineered hormone BST, which is now manufactured by Monsanto under the trade name Posilac, in cows.

BST occurs naturally in cows. The hormone stimulates milk production. Food companies, scientists and some dairy farmers reasoned that milk production could be increased if cows could be given BST supplements.

Scientists have now been able to duplicate the molecule artificially. Numerous tests have shown that the genetically engineered BST does in fact increase milk production without harming the cows. Upjohn, American Cyanimid and Eli Lilly are all planning to join Monsanto in what they think will be a lucrative market with other versions of BST.

The head of the FDA, Dr. David Kessler, who is no slouch when it comes to protecting the health of the public, says that there is no difference in the milk of cows given BST from those who have not gotten the synthetic hormone.

In announcing the agency's approval of the hormone, Kessler said that the agency "looked carefully at every single question raised and we are confident this product is safe for consumers, cows and for the environment.

Still there are many people who worry about adding milk made by cows treated with BST to the general food supply. Some have suggested that any milk that comes from cows treated with BST ought to be specifically labeled as such so that consumers would know.

Thus far, FDA officials have resisted imposing any special labeling requirements. They believe that since there is no difference in the milk made by cows given genetically engineered BST, there is no need for a special label. Milk can, however, be labeled as BST-free if dairies decide they wish to do that.

If artificially made BST-generated milk is the same as naturally occurring BST-generated milk, then what is the issue?

The unstated issue around the availability of synthetic BST to increase milk production is jobs. Small dairy farmers are especially worried that the availability of BST will put them out of business. There is already a surplus of milk in the United States. BST is likely to drive the price of milk down in an already glutted market, thereby driving out some dairy producers.

In dairy states such as Minnesota and Wisconsin, the pressure to keep BST out or at least to compel the labeling of milk made from cows given the hormone has been enormous.

But arguments to require labeling of BST-made milk in order to preserve the small dairy farmer make no sense. If science finds ways to make more food using less human labor and fewer animal sources, then agriculture is going to have to adjust to that reality. Anyone who thinks the way to save jobs in this country is by resisting technological change should take a long hard look at the American automobile and steel industries.

Milk made from cows fed with genetically engineered BST will be at your grocer's soon. Genetically engineered tomatoes and other fruits and vegetables will not be far behind. So far, the regulatory oversight that has been given to foods made through genetic engineering seems more than adequate to assure that they are safe.

BST-made milk ought to be the least of my family's worries when, next February, they see old Dad sitting down to inhale a bowl of Smackin' Good Floatin' Sugarcoated Turtlesquares.

"Gene Zoo" Proposal Deserves
More Scrutiny by Public

The Senate Committee on Governmental Affairs met on April 26, 1993 at the request of Hawaii's Sen. Daniel Akaka to listen to testimony about the Human Genome Diversity Project. This jargony title refers to a proposal by researchers to systematically sample human DNA from all of the sub-populations, ethnic groups and races now living in the world today.

Scientists such as geneticists Luca Cavalli-Sforza of Stanford University and Mary Claire King of the University of California at Berkeley think that if they can compile a thorough sample of the heredity make-up of all the various groups living in the world today, they would have an invaluable resource for understanding human origins, migration and the susceptibility to various diseases that may exist in certain groups or sub-populations.

In other words, by creating a kind of gene zoo, where a snapshot of the distribution of humankind's genetic blueprints is kept, scientists would have a repository they could use to do more of the kind of work correlating diseases and genes that led to the exciting findings on colon cancer.

Proponents think the project could be done in about five years at a cost of around $25 million. Blood samples, saliva and hair would have to be collected from roughly 25 people representing each of the 600 recognized population groups now living on Earth. In some cases this would mean sending scientists into very remote areas of the globe to obtain samples from isolated populations.

The tissues would then need to be preserved on the spot and then rushed to a central collection site. At the repository some of the samples would be stored for future research. Cells from other samples could be artificially stimulated to grow exact copies of themselves.

Researchers would then extract the DNA from these cloned cells to create a biodiversity map of humankind that could be used to better understand biological relationships among human groups and to more accurately pinpoint the role played by heredity in diseases such as cancer.

Amidst all the furor about the assault on David Koresh and his lunatic followers in Waco, Clinton's health reform plans and the struggle to bring genocide to an end in Bosnia, perhaps it is not surprising that a session on the wisdom of creating a gene museum held before an obscure Senate committee got little attention in or out of Congress.

It is not surprising, but it is inexcusable. The decision about whether or not to fund the Human Genome Diversity Project is one of the most important our society faces.

The project holds much promise, but there are real ethical dangers in trying to create a gene zoo. As Professor Henry Greely of the Stanford University Law School pointed out in testimony at the hearing, obtaining tissue samples from subjects in the remotest parts of the globe who have no understanding of DNA or genetics raises obvious questions about informed consent and the potential for exploitation.

Nor is it clear who, if anyone, would own the materials information collected by the Human Genome Diversity Project or who should be able to access the project's samples, data or findings.

Most troubling is the fact that human beings do not have an especially distinguished track record when it comes to using information about genetic differences. There is a real danger that the genetic information found by the Human Genome Diversity Project could be used to support racist or nationalist claims about "genetic superiority" or the "purity" of a particular group.

In a world where so many people die as a result of racial, ethnic, tribal and clan conflicts, more knowledge about the biological basis of human differences might be a very dangerous thing.

The proposal to undertake the Human Genome Diversity Project deserves the kind of examination that Sen. Akaka wisely tried to stimulate by convening his hearing. Despite the moral risks involved, the creation of a genetic map of humankind deserves your attention.

If Genetic Finds Win Patents,
Let NIH Hold Them

Scientists at the National Institutes of Health in Washington, D.C., have been very busy rummaging through cells obtained from a collection of human brains. By extracting the DNA from these cells, they can locate the information that permits a stew of chemicals to become a bit of brain. The NIH scientists are breaking the brain's genetic code at a rapid rate; about 180 new sequences a day. At this pace, they will have a rough map of all of the 30,000 genes expressed in human brain cells in a year.

The rapid progress being made in mapping these genes has set some other brain cells working. These are located in the heads of the lawyers, venture capitalists, Wall Street analysts, corporate executives and government officials who are wondering who will own these gene maps.

The NIH scientists were going to publish some of their initial discoveries in the prestigious journal *Science*. Just before they did, the attorneys responsible for patents at the NIH got wind of their publication plans. The lawyers realized that if the newly discovered genetic sequences appeared in print without a patent having been filed, then anyone could use them without having to pay fees or royalties. The lawyers gagged. The NIH attorneys kiboshed publication until they could file patent applications on the genetic sequences.

Many members of the scientific community were and remain outraged at the decision to seek patents on the information stored in brain cell genes. They feel that information about the genetic code ought to be freely available to anyone who wishes to use it. While morally highminded, it is doubtful whether their view can prevail. The free exchange of information may prove to be no competition when the stakes are in the tens of billions of dollars.

Big money rides on controlling knowledge about the genetic blueprints of human, plant and animal cells. The pharmaceutical, agricultural, medical and biotechnology industries in this and other countries all plan to make new products based on the emerging understanding of the genes that differentiate, at least superficially, Dan Quayle, a turnip and a toad.

Whoever controls knowledge about the genetic makeup of humans, plants and animals will have a huge edge in getting products to market.

The lawyers at the NIH know this. That is why they sought patents even though their scientists have got only a partial list of the genetic sequences in brain cells. The NIH wizards have no idea what these sequences mean. If the patent application fails it will not be on the grounds that genes cannot or should not be patented. Rather, it will fail because no one at the NIH can yet say what practical plans it has for applying this new knowledge. Demonstrating utility is one of the key requirements for getting a patent.

But the fact that no one is quite certain what to make of all this new knowledge has not stopped others from filing for patents. The Medical Research Council in the United Kingdom filed for patents on some genetic sequences discovered by British scientists. Other governments and corporations will surely follow.

We are on the verge of a microscopic version of the Oklahoma land rush. Scientists, governments and companies are about to dash out over the molecular landscape of the genes to stake their claims.

The patenting of genetic information seems inevitable. If that is so, then even though the NIH is probably a bit premature, it might be on to something important. It would best if no proprietary ownership were granted over the genetic code. Applied knowledge, rather than pure knowledge, ought to be the stuff of patents.

But if our courts are willing to let patents be granted on genetic sequences, then maybe it is better if the nation's leading scientific institution owns the code in the name of the taxpayers who foot the bill for the research. If the huge sums of money to be made from licensing the genetic code are cycled back to the NIH to fund future biomedical research, then maybe assigning patents to the NIH isn't such a bad idea.

Unearthing the Secrets
of a Longer Life

Scientists at the University of Colorado's Institute for Behavioral Genetics reported the discovery of a recessive gene that increases the mean lifespan of the species *Caenorhabditis elegans* by 65 percent. In plain English, the scientists found that when a rare genetic message is present in the eggs of roundworms, they live a lot longer than the rest of their pals.

Ain't it great! The National Institutes of Health takes your tax money and uses it to fund research to discover why some worms live longer than others.

The fact that the IRS continues to create tax forms that take longer than anyone's lifespan to complete remains beyond human understanding—but the nation is paying a gaggle of Ph.D.s to unearth the lifestyles of worms.

Well, before you dash off your letter of outrage to your favorite congressional profligate, you should know that the Colorado researchers' attempt to understand aging in the roundworm may have tremendous significance for understanding why you and I and all other living things live, age and die.

The researchers suspect that the gene responsible for setting the clock that determines how long a worm lives—which they call "age-1"—is a relatively simple, regulatory gene. If, by using some of the new techniques of recombinant DNA technology, they can locate, identify and isolate this gene, they could then look at human genes to see if an analogous form exists.

Researchers have long suspected that the changes characteristically associated with aging—graying hair, wrinkling skin, creaky joints, fragile bones, hearing loss, and so on—are, in part, controlled by heredity. The clues are everywhere: Everyone ages, but not everyone ages at the same rate. And while everyone ultimately dies, not everyone dies at the same age. Indeed, there is a very rare fatal genetic disease that causes in young children a set of changes that looks remarkably like hyper-aging.

If the genes that control our biological clocks are similar to those at work in the roundworm, we may be on the verge of unlocking the secret of a longer life. Imagine being able to reset our genetic biological clocks so that the proverbial three score and 10 is no longer the outer limit of human longevity.

If we can understand the genetic basis of aging, should we try to intervene to alter our natural limits?

Before you volunteer to be the first guinea pig, keep in mind what changing our lifespan entails. If science can slow the sands of time, we might wind up living longer, but not necessarily healthier lives. More time here might only mean more time to develop arthritis, Alzheimer's, Parkinsonism, cardiac disease or strokes.

Even if it turns out that we—or more likely, our children—could get a better chance of living longer by genetic engineering, should we take the chance? Would your kids really appreciate your helpful advice for another couple of decades? Could your spouse take another 30 years of your snoring? Would anyone younger than 80 have a shot at a promotion, tenure or a corporate dictatorship? Imagine what an "oldies" station would sound like.

Wondering whether we would try to make death take a holiday is silly. I have no doubt that if we crack the secret of aging, we will inexorably push on, regardless of the economic, cultural and social consequences, and try to extend our lifespans. But remember, even the roundworms with the lucky genetic mutation do not live forever. We may learn to delay our deaths, but we will still die.

CHAPTER 8
RATIONING AND THE DISTRIBUTION OF
SCARCE MEDICAL RESOURCES

Governor Transplant Case Shows
Real Issues of System Fairness

It wasn't long after Pennsylvania Gov. Robert P. Casey was wheeled into the operating room of Presbyterian University Hospital in Pittsburgh to receive a heart and liver transplant that the sniping started.

Americans know there are long waiting lists for those in need of transplants. They also know that many people die before an organ is found for them. So when the governor got two organs less than 48 hours after being admitted to the hospital, a lot of folks began to wonder what strings had been pulled to catapult Casey to the head of the line.

It should come as no surprise that the allocation of organs to those in need generates so much debate and discussion. The only way to get organs from the dead is if they or their next of kin altruistically donate them.

True, the occasional free marketeer economist does suggest we try bribing people to get them to make their parts available when they die. And American transplant teams do cast an envious eye toward Belgium, Austria and France, which have laws permitting organs to be taken unless there is some reason to think the deceased would have objected.

But Americans have made it clear that they believe the proper moral foundation for getting organs from those who have died is voluntary, altruistic consent. Voluntary consent works only if those who donate believe that their gifts are used fairly and equitably. If political leaders, celebrities or the rich can cut in line to get a transplant, then few Americans will be willing to check off their drivers' licenses or carry an organ donor card.

For altruism to work, the distribution of organs must be squeaky clean. The appearance of the Pennsylvania governor in a surgical suite getting two organs before many others had had a chance at one left a lot of Americans wondering if some wheels squeak louder than others where organ transplants are concerned.

Could a governor, or for that matter a senator or a president, pull strings to get a transplant? As I asked, only rhetorically, in a 1992 book of mine, *If I Were a Rich Man, Could I Buy a Pancreas?*, I don't think so.

Sure, doctors, nurses and hospital administrators know when a famous politician or wealthy person is being worked up for a transplant. No doubt, the knowledge that someone is a celebrity may lead a doctor to look extra hard at a test result or to bend over backwards to make sure that everything that can be done has been done. Doctors are no less immune to celebrity than anyone else.

But the fact that the governor of Pennsylvania wound up at the head of the list of people waiting for transplants had a lot more to do with his doctors' diagnosis that Casey was in imminent danger of dying than who he was.

Casey has a hereditary disease, amyloidosis, in which the cells in his liver produce a chemical that damages the liver and other organs. When doctors examined Casey, they found that his heart was so severely damaged that he could have died within hours. His urgent need for a transplant pushed Casey to the head of the list.

In the early '80s it was not uncommon for wealthy foreigners to pay big bucks to push their way to the head of the line for a transplant. This trade got so out of hand that Congress insisted a national system be created to ensure that Americans got first crack at the organs that became available and that organs be distributed in an equitable manner.

The United Network for Organ Sharing, based in Richmond, Va., has had Congress' mandate to keep an eye on the distribution of organs ever since. The network's policies give priority to medical urgency, along with matches in blood type, tissue type and recipient size in deciding who will get the next available kidney, heart, liver or lungs.

Current rules give organs to the sickest. Those like Casey, who might die at any moment, are first in line regardless of how long others have been waiting.

If the governor did not jump the queue, then did he get any other special favors? Yes. But these had more to do with getting into a transplant center than getting a transplant so quickly.

The governor of Pennsylvania, unlike tens of millions of other Americans, has a health insurance plan willing to cover experimental multiple organ transplants.

Many Americans needing transplants have no insurance. They are not first on any waiting lists because they do not get through the hospital door. They are told that they must raise the money necessary to pay for a transplant before they will be considered for a transplant.

The governor of Pennsylvania did not have to pull strings to zoom to the head of the line to get a transplant. His failing liver and heart did that for him.

The governor did have the advantage of his office and the generous insurance benefits it carries. The true test of the fairness of our health care system is not who is first on the waiting list. It is whether all of those who need a transplant can get onto the waiting list in the first place.

Transplants: Let's Disregard
the Differences

There has been a lot of discussion among transplant surgeons—most of it behind closed doors—about whether race should be taken into account in allocating cadaver kidneys for transplantation.

Among blacks, transplanted kidneys are somewhat more likely to fail, and the death rate after transplants is slightly higher than among whites.

No one is sure why this is so.

One factor seems to be that there are relatively fewer cadaver kidneys obtained from blacks than there are from whites, so it is harder to find biologically suitable kidneys. Since genetic and biological differences influence the success of kidney transplants, some experts think that the difference between black and white survival rates is, in part, a result of the fact that blacks who receive kidneys from whites do not do as well with them as whites do.

Other factors that may play a role in the difference between survival rates include differences in the kinds of diseases that cause kidneys to fail, the effects of the drugs necessary to prevent rejection of the kidney and differences in the levels of compliance in taking anti-rejection drugs.

Black-white survival differences have led to a heated, if quiet, debate about whether race should be taken into account when making decisions about who should receive priority for transplants. If the goal is to maximize the number of lives saved, race ought to be taken into account in deciding who should receive a transplant. If the goal is to make sure that every American has a fair shot at a transplant, race should not matter.

But before you make up your mind, consider another factor that influences transplant success rates. With a group of my colleagues when I was at the University of Minnesota, I looked at the role that weight plays in the outcome of cadaver kidney transplant. We found that transplant recipients who weigh more than 200 pounds are at a significantly higher risk of losing their kidneys than those who weigh less than 150 pounds. Regardless of age or sex, if you weigh more than 200 pounds, you are more likely to die after a transplant than someone who weighs less than 150 pounds.

The difference between the fat and the svelte in death rates and kidney loss is greater than the difference due to race. So if you thought race should be taken into consideration, you'll have to consider weight, too. If you're plump, you'll lose out to skinnier specimens of the species.

And if you're a man, which means there's a good chance that you weigh more than a woman, you'll have less of a chance of getting a transplant than a member of the lighter sex.

I think efficiency and effectiveness should be considered—but we have to be fair. We should not ask any group—black or white, fat or thin—to go to the end of the waiting line for life-saving transplants unless there is a huge difference in survival rates. There isn't. Therefore, neither size nor skin color should be used to decide who lives and who dies.

Transplant Candidate's Drug Conviction Must Not Turn into Death Sentence

DeWayne Murphy is 33 years old. There is a good chance he will not live to see 34. He is dying of heart failure. Murphy need not die. If he receives a heart transplant, there is a very good chance he will live a long life.

But Murphy is serving a four-year prison term in the federal prison in Rochester. His jailers will not let the convicted felon be evaluated by a transplant team to see if he is medically eligible to go on the waiting list for a heart transplant. In doing so, they are sentencing him to death. And that is wrong.

In October 1990, Murphy went to the doctor complaining of chest pain and shortness of breath. An examination revealed that his heart had grown to three times its normal size and was pressing up against his lungs. He had a rare mysterious condition known as cardiomyopathy in which, for reasons that are not clearly understood, the muscle of the heart irreversibly deteriorates.

Murphy was told by his doctors that he would need a transplant. Less than a year later he was arrested for possession of a large amount of methamphetamine, convicted and sent to the slammer.

OK, DeWayne Murphy did get busted for drugs. But, why won't federal prison officials let him be evaluated for a transplant? It cannot be that a heart transplant program is hard to find. The Mayo Clinic is barely a stone's throw away from Murphy's cell. Perhaps the federal authorities do not think a felon should be allowed to compete for a scarce donor heart.

The United Network for Organ Sharing, the organization in Richmond, Va., that distributes donor organs to hospitals around the nation, says that more than 2,800 people are now on its waiting list for hearts. Roughly 40 percent of those on the list will die because no organ becomes available.

But, surely it cannot be right to keep Murphy off the transplant list because he is a convicted felon. When Gov. Casey of Pennsylvania got his heart/liver transplant at the University of Pittsburgh, there was a great collective gnashing of teeth about the possibility that he had gotten ahead of others, less famous, less powerful on the waiting list. If that had happened it would have been wrong. But, it would be equally wrong to exclude the poor or the socially undesirable from their chance at life.

Murphy would not be refused the right to donate his organs because he is a convicted felon. He was sentenced to four years, not death. He has as much right to complete for a scarce donor heart as the governor of Pennsylvania or anyone else.

Maybe what is sticking in the craw of the feds is the cost of a heart transplant. The operation can run anywhere from $80,000 to $150,000 depending on how well things go. That looks like a pretty sizable chunk of change to spend on a convicted drug dealer.

It is a lot of money. But Murphy's family says he has the insurance to pay for the transplant. And even if he did not, cost should not be the driving factor in deciding whether a 33-year-old man can get access to a life-saving medical procedure of well-established efficacy.

Some might say that it is nuts to let a prisoner get a transplant when there are many Americans with no health insurance who might not be able to afford the procedure were they to need it. But the solution to that problem is not to kill DeWayne Murphy. It is to make sure that every American, even those not in prison, has access to health insurance that covers proven medical treatments.

Murphy's mother, Pat, a retired nurse, cannot believe the Feds won't let her son be considered for a transplant. She says, "If anything happens to my son ... I will sue to the nth degree for wrongful death." She is right to be angry about what prison officials are doing to her son. She also stands a good chance of winning her suit.

DeWayne Murphy cannot believe he is being blocked from getting the surgery he needs. The father of two says that if society had wanted to sentence him to death for his crime, they should have done it "in a courtroom instead of putting me in Rochester and letting me slowly wither away." He is exactly right. It may be nuts for us to foot the bill for a convicted felon to get a heart transplant. But it is the ethical thing to do.

Helmet-Free Motorcycle Riding:
A Freedom Too Costly to Society

Spring has finally arrived in Minnesota. There are a number of ways in which the natives know that this is so. The ice is finally gone from the lakes. Robins, geese and cardinals are back. And local fruitballs are riding around on motorcycles without helmets on their heads.

Like 22 other states, Minnesota does not require motorcycle drivers to wear helmets. In Minnesota, as in 18 other states, those under 18 are required to wear them. But once you get over 18, you are free to implant your dome in the pavement if you decide to take that risk.

Studies show that in states with mandatory helmet laws, nearly 100 percent of those who ride motorcycles wear them. In states without such laws, only 50 percent of riders do.

A colleague of mine, Dr. Ellen Green, has been examining the issue of motorcycle helmet laws. She and her collaborator, Linda Bosse, have come up with some pretty gruesome statistics on the human and financial costs of riding motorcycles without a helmet.

Motorcycles amount for 2 percent of all vehicles registered in the United States and for about one-half of 1 percent of all vehicle miles traveled in a given year. But they account for 7 percent of all traffic fatalities—2,394 in 1992. Of those killed, more than 80 percent did not wear a helmet.

If the helmet issue were just a matter of deciding to risk your life for the freedom of going helmetless, it could be argued that the right thing to do is to let each rider decide. But the decision to go without a helmet is not a private one.

Studies show that accidents in which a motorcycle rider survives but did not wear a helmet racks up a hospital bill that is five times more than survivors who had a helmet on. Those costs go on your insurance premiums and mine.

Those who survive with major disabling conditions from traumatic injuries to the brain cost the taxpayer in a state like Minnesota $25,000 a year for nursing home care and more than $60,000 a year if they wind up in a state hospital. These costs are almost always paid out of public programs like Medicaid.

What possible reason could there be for letting the whopping costs of riding without a helmet be borne by you and me? One of the most persuasive reasons those who oppose mandatory helmet laws give in testifying before state legislatures is that it is more dangerous to wear a helmet than not.

Critics of helmet laws say that while helmets may protect the head, their weight transfers the force of an accident to the neck. If the only thing a helmet does is wind up breaking your neck instead of your bean, then it makes no sense to require riders to wear them.

But a study published in the *Annals of Emergency Medicine* blows this myth out of the water. Dr. Elizabeth Orsay of the University of Illinois at Chicago and a team of physicians looked at data on injuries following motorcycle accidents at 28 hospitals in Illinois, Iowa, Nebraska and Wisconsin.

In the 1,153 cases they examined, there was no connection between wearing a helmet and increased risk of spinal injuries. But injuries to the head and brain were nearly three times less likely when riders wore helmets. The authors note that "because head injuries are far more common in motorcycle crashes than are spinal injuries, helmet use significantly decreases mortality of those who use them."

There is no denying the fact that making someone wear a helmet is a restriction of their freedom. But the cost of this particular freedom—in terms of both preventable disability and unnecessary health care costs—to the community is too high. Every state should require those who ride motorcycles to wear a helmet.

Ethics of Casting the First Stone: Personal Responsibility, Rationing and Transplants

Personal responsibility for one's health as played an important, if not always explicit, role in the allocation of resources for health care in the United States for many, many decades. The field of transplantation is no exception. A variety of criteria with their roots in personal responsibility, including mental status, compliance, criminal behavior, smoking, and the use of additive drugs, are and have been used for many years in making decisions about who receives access to scarce, life-saving transplants. However, these decisions are often made under the rubric of "psychosocial" contraindications to transplant. Although many transplant teams, in their weekly meetings, think it appropriate to weigh a history of felonious criminal conduct or the fact that someone is a prisoner into their allocation equation, they are much more comfortable doing so under the rubric of psychosocial suitability than personal responsibility.

Transplant teams are not alone in trying to avoid any explicit reference to personal responsibility in their rationing decisions. Historically, physicians have tried to minimize the importance of responsibility in allocating health care resources. Doctors, nurses, and other health care professionals have recognized an ethical duty to treat those who require their services regardless of how they came to have their need.

But, in recent years, an increasing number of commentators have begun to call for a change in the traditional professional ethic requiring a duty to heal regardless of the character or conduct of the patient. Many authors believe that the time has come to invoke personal responsibility as a morally relevant criterion for guiding allocation decisions in health care. Some believe physicians should take personal responsibility into account in making decisions at the bedside about who is eligible to receive treatment. Others argue that personal responsibility, although not a justifiable basis for excluding anyone from services, should play a role in physician decisions about what priority to assign those competing for the same scarce resources. More and more frequently, politicians, health policy analysts, and public health experts suggest that more weight should be given to personal responsibility for health in public policies aimed at reducing health care costs. When President Bill Clinton launched his health reform effort with his speech on September 23, 1993 to Congress, he listed personal responsibility among the six values he said should guide the effort to reform America's health care system.

The belief that certain behaviors should be grounds for disqualification for access to resources or for assigning someone a lower priority in gaining access to health care resources is not only a matter of theory. Some primary care physicians no longer accept people who smoke as their patients. Some have argued that those who abuse intravenous drugs should be denied access to surgery to repair heart valves damaged by endocarditis. Still others have assigned lower priority to smokers for access to bypass surgery. In some dialysis programs, those who are violent, abusive, or noncompliant are disqualified from treatment even if it means their certain death. Many rehabilitation programs use psychosocial assessments, including assessment of compliance and motivation, as a standard part of their eligibility determinations in placing would-be patients on their waiting lists, as well as in making decisions to terminate care.

Personal responsibility is beginning to play an explicit role in decisions about how governments allocate their overall budgets for health care. Many states and countries levy taxes on tobacco products and alcohol at least in part because they think those who indulge in the use of such products should pay society for the health costs that accrue as a result of these unhealthy behaviors. Some governments permit groups or categories of persons who engage in harmful or risky personal behavior to be charged higher insurance premiums. Public health laws have been proposed or enacted that permit the prosecution and incarceration of those whose irresponsible behavior has health consequences for others, such as the failure to stop taking narcotic drugs during pregnancy, the failure to adequately control a vicious dog, or the failure to make sure young children ride in car seats while traveling in automobiles. The more that is learned about the connection between behavior and the need for health care services and the high costs imposed by certain behaviors on the rest of society, the more physicians and policy makers seem willing to utilize personal responsibility as an appropriate criterion for allocating health care resources.

Organ transplantation occupies a key place in current debates about the moral relevance of personal responsibility for the just allocation of health care resources. Organs for transplant are scarce and so rationing is both unavoidable and omnipresent. Transplants of solid organs are expensive and require a variety of different forms of public support and subsidy. The stakes involved in transplantation are high, often life or death, raising serious public concerns about fairness and equity with respect to allocation policies. Because transplantation depends on community altruism for the supply of cadaver organs, the public and its elected officials take an especially keen interest in the equity of norms and values guiding allocation decisions in the field of transplantation.

For many years, those in the transplant community have treated alcoholism as a contraindication to various forms of organ transplantation. This has been especially true with respect to liver transplants. In part, this was a result of the fact that initial reports on liver transplantation for those who had alcohol-related liver cirrhosis suggested poor outcomes and because of fears about recidivism with respect to alcohol abuse if a transplant was performed.

Recent reports indicate that patients with chronic liver disease due to alcoholism who receive transplants do about as well in terms of survival and psychological complications as those who require liver transplant for other reasons. Nor does there appear to be a significant difference in the resources used by alcoholic and nonalcoholic recipients. Short-term survival rates for both those with alcoholic hepatitis plus cirrhosis are not greatly different from those with only chronic cirrhosis. Controlling for the age of recipients reveals that liver transplantation could be accomplished as successfully in one group as in the other.

What these findings do is force out into the open the moral issue of whether personal responsibility should be taken into consideration in allocating scarce and expensive resources. For if it is true that the cause of liver failure in adults is far less predictive of a successful outcome than other factors, such as age or comorbidity, then it can only be values, not facts, that lead many programs to continue to exclude alcoholics from access to liver transplants.

There would appear to be three moral arguments for excluding alcoholics from access to liver transplants, which might also be used to assign them lower priority should there be other potential recipients who might be equally in need of a liver transplant. First, it might be argued that those who bring harm on themselves do not merit an investment of a large share of societal resources to repair that harm. Second, some contend that those who are at high risk of causing themselves harm again in the future should be excluded from access to expensive medical interventions, such as liver transplantation. Third, some believe that it is unwise for the transplant field to permit access to those suffering from cirrhosis or hepatitis resulting from alcohol abuse, because this population is of a size sufficient to exclude nearly all other patients suffering from liver failure from access to transplants. If alcohol abusers were to make up the overwhelming majority of those receiving liver transplants, public support for the transplant field would evaporate as a result of the stigma and opprobrium many citizens feel for those who abuse alcohol.

None of these arguments is persuasive. Although it might be viewed as unfair for society to invest large amounts of resources to repair harms done as a result of personal behavior, there is no reason to single out alcohol abuse as especially worthy of punitive exclusion from important medical services. Even putting aside the much discussed question of whether alcoholism is a voluntarily chosen behavior, equity would require exclusionary policies for individuals who require medical care as a result of conduct as diverse as participation in athletics, horseback riding, failure to wear a seatbelt or helmet while operating a motor vehicle, failure to obey speed limits, failure to stop smoking, the ownership and use of a firearm, morbid obesity, employment in environments that are dangerous or stressful or, owning a large dog, a chain saw, or a swimming pool.

Although there might be a case to be made for excluding from access or assigning lower priority to those who require transplantation, this is hardly the same as excluding alcoholics on the grounds that they may drink to excess posttransplant. Moreover, the recidivism rates associated with liver transplantation are sufficiently low as to make fears of future abuse a very weak predictor of successful transplant outcomes. Some note that it may not be fair to exclude those who drink from consideration for a transplant if the primary source of donated livers are those who die as a result of alcohol abuse. Presumably, many of these people and their families would not want to exclude others who drink from consideration as candidates for receiving organs.

Finally, there may be truth to the argument that a field that serves only those who abuse alcohol risks alienating the general public. But, many fields, such as psychiatry, psychology, oncology, infectious disease and emergency medicine, to name but a few, must cope with the reality of stigma, fear, prejudice, and bias with respect to their patients. The proper response to the problem of stigma is not to exclude patients who might benefit from transplants, but to educate the public about the importance of providing fair access to those in need and to call for the redoubling of efforts to find solutions to alcohol abuse.

In the end, data are not ambivalent. Those whose livers fail as a result of alcohol abuse can do about as well as others whose livers fail for other reasons. The only moral reason for drawing a distinction about the etiology of liver failure is whether a particular disease state lessens treatment efficacy. But, as is true in many other areas of medicine, judgments of patient virtue and vice sometimes enter into the decision about who will and will not receive care. Sadly, this still seems to be true with respect to liver transplantation. As increasing emphasis is placed on the role that personal responsibility plays in health policy and resource allocation, great care will be required lest sin become one of the tests increasingly applied at the bedside to determine who will live and who will die.

The True Test of
Health Reform

You could tell when Hillary Clinton's long-awaited health-care reform plan was released by the flood of crocodile tears pouring from every suite in the insurance industry. There was a lot of yammering about the importance of preserving as much as possible the trillion-dollar Rube Goldberg machine that is our current health-care system.

Don't believe it.

Complexity and bureaucracy are essential if those now making a good living from the current system are to continue to do. The only way to increase access, lower costs and give you peace of mind about your insurance coverage is to make the system simpler.

The major reason our health-care system costs so much while covering so few is that it is built on a number of assumptions about Americans that are no longer true. The true test of health reform is whether the administration and Congress can give you a system that is in sync with the needs of a 21st-century nation. Here are the four crucial tests you should use in sorting through the tidal wave of verbiage about health reform plans.

- **Does the plan link health insurance to your job?**

    The American family no longer depends upon a breadwinner dad who has a lifetime career with one company. Many jobs, especially in the service economy, last less than a year.

    Millions of households depend on several wage earners, part-time work and moonlighting.

    When your health insurance is linked to your job, coverage is a game of musical chairs. Which employer pays, Mom's or Dad's? Which employer contributes for covering the kids, his or hers? What if the kids' parents aren't married? Job-based insurance offers third-party payers lots of opportunities to make a buck mining the fine print and ducking liability through the manipulation of red tape about how to handle joint coverage, overlapping coverage, part-time workers or subcontractors.

    Employment-based health insurance is confusing, costly and inefficient. The more it is in evidence in health reform, the more wary you should be.

- **Does reform presuppose that you will stay married for a life-time?**
  Family-based insurance lets insurers tell Americans what their families must look like. Who holds a family policy, the old dad or the new mom, the parent with money or the one with child custody? What about kids in foster care? Family-based insurance makes kids' insurance depend on deadbeat dads. Linking insurance to the traditional family structure means a system that cannot deal with the complexities of unmarried partners, interstate marriage, single moms, adoption, surrogacy and the like. If you need to be in a family to get insurance under the president's proposed reform, you need a better plan.

- **Does the reform plan assume that you are a homebody?**
  America needs a health-care system that can keep up with migrant workers, interstate truckers, college students, retirees and frequent fliers. These days, Minnesotan can get pneumonia harvesting wheat in Iowa, back pain unloading computers in Arkansas, a broken leg skiing in Wyoming, a hip replaced while wintering in Florida, an anxiety attack while at the beach on Maryland's Eastern Shore or have an asthma attack during summer study in Vermont.

    Everyone needs a personal physician, but health-care reform must do more. It must provide coverage that goes where we go. If overage is not portable, it does not go far enough.

- **Does the plan create accountability?**
  Under our current system, nobody is accountable for universal health care. Insurers and businesses have made dodging sick people the ultimate form of cost control. America has a generation of kids who need life-long special education and who will never be as economically productive as they might have been because no one is responsible for making sure pregnant women have access to prenatal care.

    Insurers use discrimination based on age, gender, genes, jobs and addresses to avoid people who need care. Businesses use buyouts, reorganizations, personnel policies and obscure federal laws to avoid insuring employees or retirees who thought they had a promise of health care. States are trading business climate for health care, lowering taxes by decreasing state assistance for people who cannot get (or afford) private insurance.

Health-care reform is the crucial test of this administration. It is an administration that says it wants to lead America into the next millennia. That vision must extend to health care. We can no longer afford a health-care system built on 19th-century views of who we are, where we work and how we live. Health reform must fit the needs of our children, not our grandparents.

Girl's Ordeal Demonstrates How Much
Better Canada's System Is

Canadian government officials are trying to deport Zahra Jessa. On July 22, 1992, they ordered her to leave the country by Sept. 22. What is remarkable about this is that Zahra Jessa is 6 years old. She is also lying in a hospital bed in an intensive-care unit.

The young American girl suffers from chronic fibrotic lung disease and can breathe only with the assistance of a mechanical ventilator.

What is even more remarkable is that the Canadians are doing the right thing. The crisis that Zahra and her family face speaks volumes about why the Canadian health care system is superior to ours and why we ought not to tolerate the one we now have.

Zahra and her mom and dad were living near Dallas in June 1990 when her lung condition flared up and she had to go to the hospital. Her parents had no medical insurance. The doctors told the family that the little girl might do better in a colder climate. So the family decided to move to Canada to stay with some relatives in Calgary.

A few months later they decided to visit other relatives in Vancouver. It was during this visit that Zahra's lung collapsed. She was rushed to the emergency room at Vancouver Children's Hospital. Unlike American hospitals where the first order of business is to establish a patient's medical status, she was simply admitted and put on a respirator.

In the words of Dodi Katzenstein, the spokeswoman for Children's Hospital, "We don't ask for an insurance card when someone is coming in with a critical emergency. When she was admitted we did not know the family history."

This statement speaks louder than all the press releases sent out in the past year by those intent on disparaging the Canadian health care system as a model for American health reform. In some hospitals in the United States, Zahra never would have made it in the door. No insurance would mean no entry.

I know this firsthand. Two years ago my son fell and severely cut his head while visiting his grandparents. My wife swept him up and drove him to the emergency room of a medium-size hospital near Philadelphia. Before anyone would even examine him to see what the extent of the damage was, she had to undergo a complete wallet biopsy. As an out-of-state family, we were not getting into that hospital and no one was going to examine my son without some demonstration of the ability to pay.

Zahra could have died for want of insurance at that very same hospital where my wife took my son. If the fact that Zahra got in to Vancouver Children's, no questions asked, is not enough to make you fervently wish for the complete overhaul of the fiasco that passes for the American health care system, then consider this: Zahra, whose family has no insurance, has now rung up bills in the amount of $1,070,000 and counting! It is expensive to stay in an intensive care unit.

Since Zahra's family has no insurance, the province of British Columbia is picking up the tab for her care under the province's universal health care insurance plan. Anybody want to take a bet on how close a 6-year-old kid with no health insurance would get to accumulating a $1 million bill in an out-of-state hospital in the United States?

But, even the Canadians have their limits. Since Zahra does not really need to be in an intensive care unit, they want to send her home. Home for Zahra is now Washington state, since her father moved there a couple of months ago when he got a new job.

The hospital officials in Vancouver figured that Zahra could go home as soon as an American hospital agreed to supervise her home care. They asked three hospitals in Dallas and three in Seattle if they would take the girl. So far all have refused. They appear to be worried about Zahra's insurance status.

Canadian officials are angry, and rightly so. They have a child from another country who does not belong in an intensive care unit, who has built up a mountain of medical bills that the province of British Columbia is paying—all because America's health care insurance situation is so bonkers that a little girl cannot find a hospital willing to accept her so that she can go back to her own country.

That is how Zahra, her mother and her 3-year-old sister come to be staring at a deportation order. Vancouver Children's Hospital President John Tegenfeldt says that, deportation order or not, the hospital is not going to shove Zahra Jessa into the street. They will not let her leave until an American hospital agrees to take her. But, Tegenfeldt adds, "Canadians should not be paying the bills. We cannot go on footing the bill because of the U.S. health-care system."

He is right. What kind of a health care system makes an involuntary exile of a 6-year-old girl with chronic lung disease? What kind of a health care system would stick another country with a million dollar bill because it cannot find a hospital willing to help so that a child can get out of the hospital and go home?

I'll tell you if you haven't figured it out by now: a system that is indisputedly inferior to Canada's. A system that cries out for drastic reform. The bloated, inefficient and callous health care system that you and I have.

Even If Legal, Insurance Caps on
Selected Illnesses are Vile

An especially odd, ethically loathsome feature of health insurance coverage in America is the emerging practice of setting a monetary cap on the amount of coverage if you get sick.

More and more insurance companies and private insurance plans are setting caps on what they will pay hospitals and nursing homes for treating particular diseases. The insurance plans are saying, in effect, that some diseases are worth paying more for than others.

Allowing insurance plans to decide which diseases are worthy of care is about as absurd a place to put moral responsibility as can be imagined. But that is the way the world of insurance currently stands.

Mark Kadinger found out about this the hard way. When the St. Paul man contracted AIDS, he learned that his union medical insurance plan would pay only $50,000 to cover the costs of AIDS-related care. His bills were higher than that.

If Kadinger had been hit by a car or struck by lightening, his insurance would have covered up to $500,000 in medical bills. But because he had AIDS, he faced going bankrupt—thanks to the cap that his insurance plan had imposed on payments to treat his disease.

The practice of limiting payments according to the type of disease someone has is inherently unfair. Why should those facing huge medical bills have to worry that their insurance will run out depending upon the nature of their illness? Are those with AIDS somehow less worthy of the same degree of coverage than someone who has Alzheimers, tuberculosis, food poisoning or a spinal cord injury? Mark Kadinger did not think so.

Before he died last Nov. 20, 1992, Kadinger asked his physician, Dr. Frank Rhame of the University of Minnesota, and the Minnesota AIDS Project to take legal actin to challenge this patently immoral insurance practice.

That is why on March 17, 1993, the University of Minnesota and the estate of Mark Kadinger filed suit in U.S. District Court in Minneapolis alleging that the health plan operated by the International Brotherhood of Electrical Workers, of which Kadinger was a member, discriminated against him by capping the amount of money he could receive to pay his AIDS-related medical bills.

The legal basis for the suit was the Americans with Disabilities Act, which was enacted by Congress last year to prevent discrimination against those with disabilities.

Since AIDS is recognized as a disability under this law, the hope is—according to Gayle Dixon, legal program coordinator for the Minnesota AIDS Project—that this first of its kind lawsuit in the nation will put "employers on notice that they cannot cap specific diseases."

While the practice of putting caps on insurance payouts by disease would seem to be inherently discriminatory and unfair, some experts doubt that the lawsuit will succeed. George Annas, a professor of law, ethics and public health at Boston University, believes that the court will rule in favor of the right of the union to use disease-specific caps in its health plan.

"It is terrible that they can do this," Annas says, "but the Americans with Disabilities Act only protects individuals against discrimination, not groups. If everyone who has AIDS or any other disease has a cap placed on what they can receive in terms of health benefits, the court is not likely to find that discriminatory."

Annas' discouraging prediction about the fate of the lawsuit is echoed by his colleague at Boston University, Wendy Mariner. Mariner notes in a recent *New England Journal of Medicine* article that health plans which self-insure are turning more and more to disease exclusions and caps as a way to contain costs. At least 18 plans have reduced or eliminated health insurance benefits for those with AIDS.

Perhaps telling everyone with AIDS or Parkinson's or Alzheimers that they cannot get the same degree of medical coverage as others whose bills are the same—but whose diseases are different—does not violate the Americans with Disabilities Act.

But it surely ought to offend every American's sense of decency and fairness to permit a health care insurance system in which a faceless, bureaucratic bean-counter with an eye on the bottom line gets to decide whether your disease is one deemed worthy of payment in full.

Rather than Villain, Technology
Could Be Health Cost Savior

Who dunnit? Who is responsible for the high cost of health care in America? Lots of suspects are being hauled into lineups in newspapers, on television and in Congress.

Some policy wonks think the evidence points toward greedy doctors, drug companies and for-profit hospitals. Inspector Hillary has fingered private health insurance companies. Other health policy detectives say it is lawyers and the ridiculous state of malpractice law in this country that are driving costs through the roof.

But lots of the health policy police think these culprits are just small fry. The Mr. Big of health care cost is, they say, technology. American health care is overflowing with technology. Transplants, bypass operations, CAT scans, laser surgery and hip replacements—these are the real villains responsible for the red ink spilling out of the Federal budget.

These cost-control cops argue that unless we get tough on technology, unless we lock up the researchers and engineers who are busy right now inventing the next generation of medical innovations, we will be in hock up to our eyeballs. Technology is the bad guy.

Phooey! It is pathetic that this line of blarney has found so many receptive ears. Technology, contrary to what so many experts and pundits say, is not public enemy No. 1 when it comes to the high cost of American medicine.

A group of Dutch physicians reports that 38 percent of Dutch general practitioners are using computer-based patient records. Of these, 70 percent no longer use any written records or charts in treating their patients.

Technology may be expensive, but it can also save money. The need for more technology and lots of it is, as the Nov. 15, 1993 issue of the *Annals of Internal Medicine* makes abundantly clear, especially pressing with respect to the use of computers in medicine.

In 1863 Florence Nightingale complained in her classic book, *Notes on a Hospital*, that "I have applied everywhere for information, but in scarcely an instance have I been able to obtain hospital records fit for any purposes of comparison. If they could be obtained ... they would show how money was being spent, what amount of good was really being done with it, or whether the money was doing mischief rather than good ..."

If the good nurse were to suddenly be transported into the average American hospital, clinic or group practice of today, she would be amazed to find that her 130-year-old lament still rings true. Medical record-keeping is still in the dark ages in America.

In the United States, fewer than 1 percent of all general practitioners use computer-based patient records. The average American hospital is still using handwritten paper copies of information that are kept on file in huge record rooms. The average American doctor cannot instantaneously call up your medical record on the office computer, but must wait for someone to find your chart from the record room.

In this country it is still possible to die or be injured as a result of bad penmanship. In the current antiquated system being used for handling information, tests are repeated, errors are made, unnecessary tests done and laboratory results misplaced because no one can find your chart.

In a related article in the same issue of the *Annals*, three physicians in the Laboratory of Computer Science at the Harvard Medical School offer what is truly a horrifying diagnosis of the pathetic state of record-keeping and information storage in American medicine today. They complain of fragmented patient medical records and say, "The primary emphasis has not been on the clinical record but functions such as billing ..."

What the doctors are saying is that our current health care system is great at using computers to track you down and make sure you pay your bill, but has no idea how to use them to keep track of the state of your health.

Florence Nightingale was right. A key strategy for controlling health care costs is to use information efficiently and effectively. We are not going to get a handle on the cost of health care until President Clinton's health security card gets a spot on it for a computer chip that has your medical history encoded on it and a computer at your doctor's office that can read it. Spending money on this kind of technology not only will save money; it might even save your life.

Depo-Provera Price-Gouging
Illustrates Industry Habit

The pharmaceutical industry in the United States is getting away with extortion. The latest example of how drug companies rip off the public is the Upjohn Company's decision to jack up the price of Depo-Provera.

Depo-Provera has been on the market for some time as a cancer drug. It cost $12 a dose. In October, 1992, the Food and Drug Administration cleared Depo-Provera for use as an injectable contraceptive. Upjohn quickly raised the price to $34 a dose.

Since a woman using Depo-Provera as a method of contraception needs to get an injection about once every three months, that works out to a yearly cost of about $134. It is curious that the new price set for Depo-Provera works out to roughly what women are already used to paying for a year's worth of birth control pills.

Upjohn officials justified their price-gouging by arguing that the company is entitled to recoup their costs for the research and development that resulted in a new contraceptive option for women. But this is sheer sophistry.

The bulk of the research done on the value of Depo-Provera as a contraceptive was done many years ago. The drug has been used as a contraceptive in many nations for decades. There is no reason for suddenly jacking up the price other than that the company knows what women who use existing contraceptive drugs are already used to paying.

The story of Depo-Provera is just one element in an incredible tale of profiteering, greed and avarice. The Senate Special Committee on Aging reported in 1991 that during the 1980s, when the general rate of inflation rose by 58 percent, prescription drug prices rose a whopping 152 percent. A prescription that cost the average American $20 in 1980 cost $53.76 in 1991.

If those numbers don't make you want to take an aspirin, try these reported in a September 1992 report from the same Senate committee for drugs sold in the outpatient pharmacy of a large urban hospital:

- The price of insulin made by E.I. Lilly rose from $5.05 a dose in 1990 to $7.25 in 1991, an increase of 44 percent.
- Captopril, a heart drug made by Bristol-Myers, cost 61 cents in 1990 and 85 cents in 1991, an increase of 39 percent.

- Albuterold inhalant for asthma made by Glaxo cost $3.50 in 1990 and $5.95 in 1991. Glaxo enjoyed a 70 percent increase in one year.

Lest you think the appetite for ridiculous profits has been sated, consider what it will cost you if you need to get a year's worth of Merck's new drug Proscar for your prostate cancer—$1,095. Astra's new drug Foscavir for viral eye infection runs $21,000 a year. A single dose of Centoxin, a new antibiotic, will set back you or your insurance company a minimum of $3,000.

If you suffer from migraines, Glaxo's new drug Sumatriptan might help but only if you are prepared to shell out $100 per shot. A dose of the Nova company's new treatment for leukemia, Pergamid, will probably be in the neighborhood of $1,100.

Whenever these numbers are questioned, the pharmaceutical industry starts to huff and puff that the cost of providing a wide variety of choices of medicines and drugs is not cheap. Moreover, they say, drug prices only account for a tiny fraction, under 2 percent, of the overall amount Americans spend on health care.

It is true that it is very expensive to bring a new drug into the market. And it is also true that getting a handle on drug prices is not going to do much to slow the overall health care cost juggernaut.

But no other nation in the world gets stuck with a tab anywhere near the size of the one we pay. We pay 62 percent more for the same drugs than a Canadian would pay and 50 percent more than the average European. There is no reason why except that these other nations regulate the prices of drugs and we do not. We are simply paying too much for our medicine.

Nicotine Patch Funding Woes
Show Priority Disorder

The question came as soon as I got into the taxi taking me back home from the airport. Bill, a driver who likes to gab, could barely contain himself.

"Notice anything different about the cab?" he asked. I did not know what he was talking about. He could see that I was stumped, but my stupidity didn't faze him in the least.

"It doesn't smell smoky in here any more!" He was right. The cab no longer smelled like the junior high men's room of my youth.

Bill went on to tell me that he decided he had had it with waking up his wife at night with his hacking coughing. He finally decided to follow his doctor's advice and quit his three-pack-a-day, 40-year-old smoking habit.

His doctor had told him about nicotine patches, something that could be worn on his arm that would get enough nicotine into him to make it easier to quit. Bill had decided to try the patches. Much to his surprise, they worked. He hadn't had a smoke in four months.

I asked Bill if he had completely lost his craving for cigarettes. He said that with the patch on his arm he was not tempted to smoke, even when driving the cab, the toughest place for him to lay off the cigs.

Bill's smoke-free cab and lungs seemed to me to be one of the quiet little triumphs of public health. At least they did until I read a recent news report saying that federal officials in charge of the Medicaid program, the health insurance program for poor Americans, are considering restricting or even eliminating coverage for the costs of nicotine patches.

Individual nicotine patches are not all that expensive. Bill, who has bought a lot of them, says they go for about $2 each. But those who are on the patch need to use one every day. So, over the course of a year you're looking at costs of more than $700.

Since there are a lot of smokers who are trying the patch, and potentially millions more who might, small individual costs add up fast. Somewhere between $500 million and $700 million will be spent in the United States this year on nicotine patches.

The total costs are large enough to make companies such as Ciba Geigy that sell patches very happy, and insurance companies and government programs that face getting stuck with the bill very sad.

The patches pose an especially costly burden to state Medicaid programs, since smokers are more often poor than rich. In Oregon, for example, according to the *Oregon Health Forum* newsletter, the state Medicaid program paid out $14,294 for 94 prescriptions in January of this year. By May the Medicaid program was forking out $120,471 for 1,324 prescriptions.

Those who run Oregon's Medicaid program worry that the state is facing a $2 million bill for nicotine patches for 1992 in a budget that is already stretched to the breaking point.

The financial burden of nicotine patches is so intimidating to cost-conscious health officials that at least seven states—Minnesota, California, Alabama, Arkansas, Iowa, Idaho and Kentucky—have already decided their Medicaid programs will not pay for them.

Two million bucks is a lot of money for a strapped state program to fork out to get rid of a bad habit. But the total cost of paying for diseases caused by smoking, fires resulting from careless smoking, lost time from work, and pollution from smoke and ashes runs into the tens of billions of dollars each year.

Deciding not to pay a tab of $700 million because it costs too much while staring at a bill for smokers that is likely to be more than 10 times as large seems a little short-sighted.

In order to know whether paying for patches in both public and private insurance is worthwhile, we need to know whether they work. Putting aside Bill the Taxi Driver's personal testimonial, the fact is that good information as to whether those who use the patches really kick the smoking habit is not yet available.

Some experts believe that more than 75 percent of those who quit smoking by using nicotine patches are puffing away again within six months. Other experts think the success rate associated with the patch is higher—in the 30 percent range.

It is safe to guess that the patch does not work for everybody. But it does work for some folks such as Bill. It seems absurd not to budget money for patches even if only a quarter of those who smoke kick the habit. After all, the same rule that little numbers can add up to a big one applies to the cost of smokers.

A 25 percent success rate may not seem like much. But in a nation in which tens of millions of people still smoke, a quarter of a very big number is still a very big number. A health care system that will pay the costs of a lung transplant but won't pay for a patch to help people stop smoking is a health care system that needs to get its priorities in better order.

Don't Blame the Dying Elderly
for Health Care Cost Crisis

There is no agreement about what to do about the nation's hemorrhaging health care bill. But there is a broad consensus about why health care in America costs as much as it does.

In health policy discussions all around the country, those in the know about health policy quietly repeat the insiders' mantra—America spends too much money for expensive medical care on old people who are terminally ill.

The media have reinforced the belief that grandparents who are unwilling to shut off their respirators are the cause of our health care system's fiscal woes. Story after story flits across the screen or appears on our doorstep about how much money we spend on older Americans who are in the last year, month or day of life.

While they are not always willing to say so in public, a large number of health policy gurus believe that if the health care system could only persuade all Americans to fill out a living will or advance directive indicating that aggressive treatment ought to be stopped when the prognosis is hopeless, America would no longer face a health care cost crisis.

Sadly, the movement to encourage the use of living wills has as much to do with hopes for cost-containment as it does self-determination.

An interesting article in the April, 1993 *New England Journal of Medicine* casts doubt on whether those in the know really know what they are talking about when it comes to the reasons for the high cost of health care.

James D. Lubitz and Gerald F. Riley, who are both at the Health Care Financing Administration in Baltimore, the outfit that runs the federal Medicare program, believe the figures about the cost of health care for those in the last year of life are often misinterpreted or exaggerated.

Their study of the cost of medical treatment of those over age 65 in the Medicare program between 1976 and 1988 raises some very tough questions for those who think we can work our way out of the health care cost crisis by rationing care for the terminally ill elderly.

Lubitz and Riley report that the annual number of Medicare beneficiaries went from 23.4 million in 1976 to 29.1 million in 1988. The number of those who died remained relatively stable during this time period.

What is interesting is that despite the fact that the cost of the Medicare program skyrocketed from 1976, when the program cost $15 billion, to $73 billion in 1988, the percentage of the total spent on those in the last year of their life stayed the same.

In 1976, 28.2 percent of all Medicare expenditures went to elderly people in the last year of their lives. In 1988 the number was 28.6 percent.

This means that whatever is causing medical bills to go through the roof, it is not spending more and more on people in their final days.

Not only has the percentage of money spent on hospital care for those in the final year of life not grown in 12 years, Lubitz and Riley found that the amount of money spent on hospital care for Medicare recipients who nevertheless died actually was lower if the person died at an older age.

In 1988 the hospital bill for the last year of life for those who died at ages 65-69 was $15,436. But the bill for someone who died at ages 80-84 was $12,838. And if you were over 90 when you reached your final year on this planet, your bill was $8,888. So, the costliest Medicare patients in terms of those who ultimately die are not the oldest.

Those responsible for fixing the health care system need to pay close attention to the Lubitz and Riley findings.

The answer to the problem of cost containment is not going to be as simple as figuring out how to cut back on hospital care for the oldest, terminally ill patients. To find the right answers, we are going to have to rid ourselves of some mythology about why health care in America costs so much.

Florida's "Titanic" Plan Sank, But It Raised Elder Care Issues

Jan. 15, 1993 was a landmark day in American health policy. On that day, Florida Gov. Lawton Chiles rejected a plan that would have made his state the first in the nation to explicitly use age to ration access to health care.

In many counties in Florida, the demand for services has stretched county health department budgets to their limit. To deal with the crisis, Florida's Department of Health and Rehabilitative Services proposed a rule under which people 65 and over would have been given low priority for getting care at county health departments and clinics.

Pregnant women and children, with incomes under the federal poverty level, would have had first dibs on government-sponsored health care. Older Floridians would get in the clinic door only if children and pregnant women had already gotten their care.

The idea of favoring the young over the old quickly got labeled the "Titanic plan" because it put women and children on the health care lifeboat first. The name fit because the plan sank almost as fast as the boat.

Florida is a state with a high percentage of elderly citizens. And they do not take kindly to being told to wait to board the health care lifeboat.

Bentley Lipscomb, the head of the Florida State Department of Elder Affairs, quickly let it be known that he thought the Titanic plan ought to be torpedoed.

When, after heavy lobbying, the governor decided not to let the rule be implemented, Lipscomb said that, while he understood the fiscal constraints on the county health departments and the needs of kids, he did not think "the solution is to pull the plug on the elderly in Florida."

A spokeswoman for the governor, Julie Anbender, added that "the rejection of this policy sends a strong signal that we would discourage communities from using any policy that would exclude an entire group of people."

The governor's decision to backpedal away from his own administration's plan to ration care for the elderly makes political sense. Kids don't vote. Older people do. But it makes little ethical sense. Nearly all elderly people in Florida are covered by Medicare.

True, despite having this coverage, many either do not have ready access to a doctor or are stuck with doctors who do not accept Medicare patients because the doctors think government reimbursement rates are too low. The county health department may be the only place for Grandpa to go for a flu shot or for Grandma to go if her arthritis flares up.

Still, the first priority of county health departments ought to be to provide care for poor children and pregnant women. Medicare exists to handle the health care problems of older Americans. The elderly do not belong in county clinics, especially if their presence takes away resources from kids.

If there are problems in getting care for the elderly, then the solution is to do battle with the medical establishment and the government, not to occupy spaces in public clinics that are meant for children.

The proposal to ration care by age is startling only because it got as far as it did. While some will conclude that ideas like the Titanic plan show just how vulnerable the elderly are, I would suggest its defeat proves the opposite. The elderly can take care of themselves just fine in the political arena.

The moral challenge for older Americans is to make sure their health care needs are met without tapping the meager budgets allotted for other vulnerable members of society.

CHAPTER 9
THE ETHICS OF EXPERIMENTATION

O'Leary Calls Nation to Account in
Medical Experiment Scandal

President Clinton's secretary of energy, Hazel O'Leary, did two very courageous things in the last week of December, 1993.

Ignoring the protests and warnings of some of her top advisers, she directed that the Energy Department release the records of the Atomic Energy Commission concerning a variety of experiments done without the consent or knowledge of human subjects.

Then, in a decision that will forever secure her a place in the bureaucrat's Hall of Moral Fame, she said if Americans had been injured or killed as a result of these experiments, Uncle Sam should be fiscally responsible for any harm done.

Fessing up to wrongdoing, even wrongdoing that is decades old, in your own department is not likely to endear O'Leary to the spin doctors and risk managers of the Clinton administration or Congress. Going the next step and declaring that government ought to be prepared to compensate those it has harmed means that O'Leary had better prepare herself for a lot of lonely nights as she is scratched off the A-list for Washington parties and banquets.

What exactly did the government do in the late 1940s and 1950s that led the courageous energy secretary to stand up for what is right?

The malfeasance is very grave. Top government officials at the Atomic Energy Commission, NASA and the Public Health Service approved of experiments in which unsuspecting American soldiers were exposed to high doses of radiation, prisoners in Oregon and Washington state received large doses of radiation and compulsory vasectomies, retarded children were fed food laced with radioactive iron and calcium, seriously ill patients were given trace amounts of plutonium in doses known to be high enough to cause harm, medical students and hospital patients were injected with radioactive iron and chrome and newborn boys in four states were injected with weak doses of iodine 131, a radioactive isotope, without the explicit permission of their parents.

In nearly all of these studies, informed consent was not obtained or, when it was, the true nature of the research was not fully disclosed.

How could American government officials have sanctioned these experiments? How could researchers from such elite schools and institutions as M.I.T., Battelle Pacific Northwest Laboratory, the University of Tennessee and the University of Washington have gotten involved with such patently immoral research?

Remember, these experiments were begun at a time when the testimony from the Nuremberg trials concerning the horrible experiments performed by German scientists and doctors on unwilling and uninformed subjects at the direction of the German government and military forces was still ringing in the world's ears.

Didn't anyone take seriously the Nuremberg Code, issued by American judges at the conclusion of these trials, that made informed consent an absolute, inviolate requirement for all research involving human subjects?

The answer as to how this mess happened is war—or, more accurately, the threat of war.

At the end of World War II, American military officials were desperate for more information on the effects of exposure to high doses of radiation. They thought the chances were high that we would be involved in a nuclear war with the Russians, or, later, the Chinese.

Our government wanted to know how fast radioactive substances would be cleared from the human body and how much damage a brief exposure to high amounts of radioactivity would cause.

It was the Cold War that led researchers to expose the reproductive organs of state prisoners to high doses of radiation and to direct esteemed scientists to slip radioactive mickeys into the bodies of gravely ill patients.

When the German scientists were put on trial for the crimes they had committed in the name of medical research in the concentration camps, many said they had done so because Germany was at war. They said that the normal rules governing human experimentation had to be put aside when the nation's security was at stake.

We hung some of those men and sentenced others to prison on the grounds that those excuses did not wash. They don't.

That is why Secretary O'Leary is right to call this nation to account for its own hypocrisy with respect to the ethics of human experimentation and to argue that we now must do what we can to make whole those who rights were sacrificed in the name of national security.

Troops Should Not Be
Drug Guinea Pigs

Americans serving in our armed forces in the Persian Gulf face many risks—and there is nothing that can be done about most of them. Simply training in such an unforgiving environment already has cost scores of lives. War over Kuwait means risking tens of thousands more.

There is, however, one risk that our soldiers in the gulf should not be forced to face: biomedical experimentation.

In October, 1992, the Department of Defense asked the Food and Drug Adminis-tration to allow the use of untested vaccines and experimental drugs for troops that are the victims of a biological or chemical attack—without getting individual consent first. The FDA issued the requested waiver in December, and it becomes effective Sunday. After that date, commanders will be able to order their troops to take untested drugs and vaccines if war has broken out or if there is a "threat of combat."

Iraq has both the capacity and the will, as the Kurds of Iraq can attest, to kill using chemical weapons. Western experts on the Iraqi military think they possess missiles loaded with deadly botulism and anthrax microbes.

The Pentagon is trying to protect our troops from these horrid forms of attack. The best protection known is the use of such barriers as gas masks and protective clothing to prevent contact with the microbes or gases. However, vaccines may work against some diseases, and certain drugs may help control or reverse the symptoms in those people who have been exposed to deadly gases or incapacitating biological agents.

But it is illegal to use federal money to engage in biomedical experimentation on competent human beings without their informed consent. No exception to this policy has ever been granted. Should the threat of biological or chemical warfare in the Persian Gulf be used to allow such an exception?

No.

Yes, war is a morally unique situation. Yes, it is silly to insist that in the midst of combat no exceptions be made to the principle of informed consent. Once exposed, the only hope a soldier may have is an experimental drug. In combat, consent is neither feasible nor sensible.

But the moral situation is different outside the context of combat. Troops waiting in the field certainly can be asked whether they want to take the risk of trying an untested vaccine against botulism or Q fever. Since no one knows whether the vaccines will work or what the long-term side effects might be, there is no excuse for not getting informed consent from each soldier.

The question of consent prior to the use of experimental vaccines or drugs is one that may not be confined to our soldiers in the desert. Terrorists may try to use biological or chemical agents against civilians in the Middle East, Europe—and even the United States. One of the horrors of modern war is that everyone is a potential target.

Within reason, our military should extend to its troops the same right that you and I enjoy to choose whether to participate in biomedical experimentation. The defense of freedom is, after all, one of the main reasons why our armed forces are in the gulf. The threat of war should not be used as an excuse to ignore free choice where medical experimentation is concerned.

Vets' Test-Related Complaints Must Be Treated Seriously

The hearing room in the Dirksen Senate Office Building was jammed, not an open seat to be found. As Sen. Jay Rockefeller, D-W. Va., called the hearing to order, four men moved to the chairs arrayed before the members of the Senate Veterans' Committee.

The stories they told to the committee in May of 1994 raise serious doubts about our government's moral commitment to those who serve in the armed services of this nation. The men all had been involved in one way or another with chemical or biological warfare. They had all tested or used equipment, drugs or vaccines intended to provide protection against the deadly effects of such weapons.

One veteran of World War II, Rudolph Mills of Virginia, told of being ordered into a pressurized chamber shortly after enlisting in the Navy in April 1945.

His assignment was to breathe mustard gas as part of a test of a new type of gas mask. The mask did not work right. The gas got into Mills' throat. He subsequently lost most of his voice box and is suffering from cancer.

Another man, Earl Davenport of Tooele, Utah, worked testing protective clothing against various biological weapons at the Dugway Proving Ground in Utah. He had been accidently contaminated by toxic nerve gas. He now suffers from serious lung disease.

Lt. Colonel Neil R. Tetzlaff had been given tablets of a substance known as pyrigostine bromide when ordered to the front lines during Operation Desert Storm. This drug, while widely used to treat those suffering from muscle disease known as myasthenia gravis, had not been proven effective against an attack by nerve gas. When Tetzlaff talked with me just before the start of the hearing, he could not stop his body from shaking.

A fourth man, the Rev. Dr. Barry Walker, who served with the Quartermasters group during Desert Storm, had been given shots of Botulanism pentavalent antitoxoid to protect him against possible biological weapons attack.

The Department of Defense was afraid the Iraqi army would break international covenants and agreements and use biological weapons as part of its Scud missile attacks. But the effectiveness of this vaccine was not certain. And those who ordered the shots be given knew there were possible side effects.

Walker told the senators that ever since his exposure, he had a lot of mysterious ailments. He also said that he had personally tried to help more than 150 other soldiers, many sitting in uniform in the hearing room, who had suffered from various maladies and problems as a result of their service in the Gulf.

Each of these men said that they wanted to serve their country. They were adamant about the fact that if called upon they would do so again. But they felt that their country had not been fair to them.

They complained that they were not getting help for their medical and psychological problems from the Veterans Administration hospital system. They said that they faced a sea of red tape when they made claims for service related disabilities.

Sen. Tom Saschle, D-S.D., himself a Vietnam War vet, seemed especially ticked off at the lame performance of the Department of Defense, the Veterans Administration and the armed services in responding to the health care problems of veterans.

"Is it not time," he asked one VA official, "to shift the burden of proof faced by those seeking treatment and compensation for service related disabilities from the veteran to the government?"

If ever there was a group that had the right to expect that their health care problems would be greeted with a sympathetic ear and a willingness to go the extra mile, it is veterans. We have created a special right to health care for those who serve and are injured as a result of that service. And we have created a health care system, the VA, with a budget bigger than the entire British National Health Service, to afford that right.

Yet, as the hearing made painfully clear, all too often the claims of veterans for treatment are greeted with hostility, suspicion and just plain arrogance. The knowledge that someone may try to shoot a shell filled with anthrax at your head may make the risks of getting a shot in your arm to protect against such weapons seem piddling by comparison. But, when military personnel are given new, investigational or unproven drugs and vaccines or agree to test protective gear in dangerous experiments, they have the right to expect that their health will be closely monitored, that any problems will be quickly diagnosed and that they will receive expeditious treatment. For too many veterans, that right is an empty promise.

Medical Research Can't Accommodate
"Abnormal" Women

Women are the victims of discrimination in medical research. Men are overrepresented in tests of new drugs, devices and procedures.

The lack of women in research is a serious problem. Drugs and devices tested only on men may turn out to have dangerous, even lethal, complications when given to women. And if testing is skewed toward the problems of men, then the health-care needs of women may be overlooked or underestimated.

Those in the federal government responsible for funding biomedical research have been told to make sure that more women are used as research subjects. Those looking for an answer to the problem are treating participation in research on a par with problems of gender discrimination in pay and employment.

It is not quite right to say that men outnumber women in biomedical research. Young and middle-aged men outnumber other participants. And these men are likely to be relatively healthy, since many research studies explicitly exclude anyone with disabilities, psychosocial problems or chronic illnesses.

The problem of the underrepresentation of women in research is real, but it is not unique. What is unique are the reasons why women are not involved to the same extent as young or middle-aged men. The key reasons: babies and ovaries.

Women have traditionally, intentionally and explicitly been excluded from biomedical research for fear that drugs, chemicals and medical devices of unknown safety and efficacy might be especially dangerous to an embryo or fetus.

Women, the common wisdom of research has long maintained, do not always know if they are pregnant and, in some cases, do not care. Drugs or radiation that are slightly risky for adults can be very risky for a developing embryo. The safest course for protecting embryos—and for protecting against lawsuits that might come in the wake of deformed or stillborn babies born to mothers involved in medical research—is to exclude them.

Paternalism toward fetuses and condescension toward women regarding their ability to be responsible about their reproductive status partially accounts for the absence of women from medical research. But these attitudes are not going to be changed by imposing the equivalent of an affirmative-action program for recruiting female research subjects.

The other reason why researchers have steered away from women is that they have ovaries. Thus they experience ovulation, menstruation, pregnancy and menopause—phenomena that predominantly male researchers view in a negative light.

For centuries, male scientists and physicians have seen men as representing and illustrating what is normal and healthy about human beings. Male physiology and behavior define normal human physiology and behavior. Women, as a number of feminist scholars have been pointing out for many years, are seen as "deviations." Since scientists want to conduct research with subjects who are as normal, as "typical" as possible, bias against non-male traits leads to the exclusion of women as suitable subjects.

Ordering those who fund science to fix gender discrimination by quota or by fiat won't work. Unless the biomedical community begins to take serious the idea that women are just as normal as men, researchers will continue to be wary of using them as research subjects. And unless society debates and reaches consensus on ethical, legal and social policies that ought to govern involvement of pregnant women and women of child-bearing age in research, researchers will continue to steer away from these women.

Discrimination against women in research will not end until doctors, scientists and legislators agree that it is normal to be female.

Safeguards Must Remain Stringent in
Trials of Experimental Drugs

On Sept. 1, 1993, a 37-year-old woman died at the University of Virginia Medical Center. She had spent the previous two months in an intensive-care unit after receiving two liver transplants.

Sometimes liver transplant surgery doesn't work. And it is not at all unusual for a second liver transplant to fail. But what was especially troubling about the death of this woman is that she died because she was a participant in a medical experiment.

Her death is a grim reminder that medical research can be dangerous, even deadly, for those who choose to participate. Her death is also a warning that calls to weaken or eliminate FDA and federal regulations about who gets experimental drugs should be viewed with great skepticism.

The woman from Virginia died while taking an experimental drug called Fialuridine or FIAU. Four other subjects have also died. Another is still in the hospital. Two others have been recently discharged after undergoing emergency liver transplants.

How did this sad state of affairs come to pass?

Scientists originally became interested in FIAU in 1989 when they noticed that patients with AIDS did better when given the drug.

FIAU did nothing to kill HIV, the virus that causes AIDS. But some of those with AIDS also had a viral disease in their livers—hepatitis. The AIDS researchers were astounded to see that subjects who got small doses of FIAU had no traces of the hepatitis B virus in their bodies after only a few days on the drug.

Hepatitis is a serious health problem in its own right. The virus slowly damages the liver, and that progressive damage, after many years, can cause liver failure or liver cancer.

Hepatitis is much more contagious than AIDS. More than 300 million people worldwide are infected with the hepatitis B virus. In the United States, more than a million people have acquired the virus through blood transfusions, sexual intercourse, needle sharing or other behavior involving the exchange of blood or bodily fluids.

Researchers at the National Institutes of Health in Bethesda, Md., were so excited by FIAU's ability to kill the hepatitis virus that, in cooperation with officials at Eli Lilly & Co., the drug's manufacturer, they organized an experiment to test the drug in humans who had hepatitis but not AIDS.

Twenty-four volunteers took small doses of FIAU for 28 days during April 1992. Again, the drug wiped out the hepatitis B virus. While two subjects had some complications, the researchers did not believe that they were the result of taking FIAU.

So the decision was made to undertake a test using a bigger dose of FIAU for a longer period of time. Volunteers with hepatitis B were recruited. They were to take FIAU for six months.

Tests showed no virus present in their bodies. But in early June, several subjects began to complain of nausea and loss of appetite. By the end of June, the experiment turned into a disaster. Two subjects had been admitted to hospitals with life-threatening problems. The NIH researchers called all of the subjects to order them to stop taking FIAU.

Dr. Jerry Hoofnagle, a hepatitis expert who ran the NIH study, told the *Los Angeles Times* that the complications were due to the fact that FIAU was poisoning the mitochondria of the cells in those who took the drug.

Mitochondria are like tiny motors that create the energy every living thing requires for life. Viruses have them, and FIAU shuts them down, causing the hepatitis B viruses in each volunteer to die. But FIAU was also interfering with the mitochondria in the cells of each subject's liver, kidney and pancreas. In larger doses, the drug was toxic to both viruses and healthy cells.

Those agreed to participate in the study to test FIAU probably never imagined that the drug might cost them their lives. These days, most of us tend to think the difference between therapy and research is just a matter of which word you prefer to use. The FIAU tragedy shows that research and therapy are not at all the same.

While both have risks, the risks of therapy are known. The risks of experiments with new drugs are not. If experimentation with human beings is to be ethical, those who volunteer to serve need to clearly understand the difference.

Using Pig Livers in Transplants Is
Building a Bridge to Nowhere

For the past 25 years, I have spent Christmas at my in-laws. They live in the town of Delran, N.J., just outside Philadelphia. For a good number of those years, a major topic of discussion around the dinner table was whether the Betsy Ross Bridge would ever be finished.

The bridge links North Philadelphia to southern New Jersey. For a long time, however, the span stood incomplete. The Betsy Ross started near Delran and crossed the Delaware River, but like some huge, weird outdoor art object, ended suspended in mid-air somewhere over the Fishtown neighborhood of Philadelphia. Many bets were made over the Stojak Christmas ham about when if ever the "bridge to nowhere" would be completed.

I've been thinking a lot lately about the Betsy Ross Bridge as a result of the decision by a team of surgeons at Cedars-Sinai Medical Center in Los Angeles to try to save the life of a 26-year-old woman, Susan Fowler, by giving her a pig liver transplant. The surgeons said that they took this desperate measure because they were "faced with a young woman deteriorating in front of our eyes with signs of severe brain swelling."

Dr. Leonard Makowka and his transplant team felt that Fowler was at death's door. They did not think she would survive long enough to get a liver from a human donor. So they decided to use the pig's liver to hold her over, to provide a bridge, until a human liver could be found.

When the subject turns to the use of animals as sources of organs for transplants, the issue that dominates debate is the morality of killing animals to save people. This is unfortunate, especially when the animal is a pig.

I have nothing against pigs. As someone who has wandered around a State Fair or two, I know pigs are relatively bright animals who have gotten a bad rap because of their proclivities with mud. But those who want to protect pigs would do them much more good if they devoted their efforts toward diminishing their presence at breakfast. If the moral choice is whether to save a pig or a human life, there is no doubt in my mind that porcine interests must yield to people's.

The real ethical questions about using a pig liver as a bridge to a human liver transplant concern humans, not pigs. Was the process of consent adequately handled by the group at Cedars-Sinai? Does the current state of knowledge about pig transplants support efforts to use them? And does the use of a pig liver as a bridge to tide someone over until a human live becomes available make good ethical sense? I would answer "no" to each of these questions.

By the time Susan Fowler was considered for a pig liver transplant, she had become comatose. Consent for the procedure was obtained from her family and the hospital's ethics committee. But the transplant team must have known for some time that they might try to use a pig liver to hold over a dying patient. The idea of trying a pig transplant as a bridge did not suddenly occur to them. While Fowler's emergency was all too real, it was an emergency that is easy to anticipate. People die every day because there are no human livers to give them. If the thing to do is tide some or all of them over with a pig's liver, then these plans ought to be made known to the medical community and to the patient long before they become comatose.

The scientific case for trying a pig liver transplant is weak. There have been relatively few published studies in the professional, peer-reviewed literature of medicine on transplants using pig livers in other animals, much less people. The state of knowledge about the use of animal organs in humans, especially non-primate organs, is so poor that almost every transplant surgeon I have asked thinks that trying a pig liver transplant in a human being at the present time is at best reckless.

Suppose the experts are wrong. Breaking new ground sometimes means bucking popular opinion. Suppose a pig liver might work just long enough to tide someone like Susan Fowler over until she could get a human liver. The fact is that using a pig liver as a bridge when human organs are so scarce is likely to cost more lives than the strategy saves. A human liver was diverted from UCLA to Cedars-Sinai for Susan Fowler, but she died before it could be used. The human liver was sent back to UCLA and transplanted in another patient.

Is it fair for a scarce human liver to go first to someone who is comatose, imminently dying and has just had a pig liver transplant, or should it go to someone who stands a better chance of living by getting the organ? Sadly, the supply of human organs is so scarce that, despite the good intentions of the doctors at Cedars-Sinai, using a pig liver is like building a bridge to nowhere.

Baboon-Liver Transplant Raises
Ethical Issues

A 35-year-old man dying of liver failure received a transplant on June 29, 1992.

There is nothing especially newsworthy about that, since there are more than 2,000 liver transplants performed each year in the United States.

What was remarkable was that the liver came from a baboon. This was the first attempt to use a liver from a baboon in a human recipient. So far, the transplant seems to be going well.

While it is still too early to say that the experiment is a success, it is not too early to examine the morality of this experiment with a baboon liver.

Most of the ethical commentary that accompanied the experiment has focused on the question of the morality of killing a baboon to save a human life. But, is there really a moral issue about the propriety of killing a baboon to save a person?

Perhaps it is morally wrong to kill animals to eat them, for sport or for their furs. But can anyone take seriously the idea that we ought to flip a coin in weighing the moral value of a baboon and a human?

People are moral agents; baboons are not. If one must die to save the other, that may be tragic, but the choice of whom to sacrifice seems clear.

More vexing, if less widely discussed, are the questions of whether the time had come to try this experiment in a human being and, if so, what the overall aim is of such research. Even if the experiment works and the patient survives with a reasonable quality of life, it still is not clear that the Pittsburgh experiment should get unqualified passing ethical grades.

The surgeons at Pittsburgh gave two reasons to justify their decision to try using an animal transplant, or xenograft. The recipient of the baboon liver, who continues to request anonymity, is infected with hepatitis B. This virus was responsible for the destruction of his liver.

The doctors in Pittsburgh said the man probably would not have been eligible for a human cadaver liver transplant due to his hepatitis, and that the odds of the hepatitis virus reinfecting a new liver, if he somehow got one, were low.

Are these reasons persuasive?

When the baboon liver transplant was being done, I was in Strasbourg, France at an international conference of experts in xenografting. Some of the surgeons there said that they would accept into their programs patients dying from liver failure as a result of hepatitis. A few of the surgeons and scientists who were there expressed skepticism about whether or not a baboon liver was vulnerable to hepatitis infection, but many thought the odds were probably lower.

The only way to know whether baboon livers are vulnerable to destruction by human hepatitis virus is to infect them. And the only way to know whether a transplanted baboon liver can do what a liver is supposed to do in another species is to transplant some.

But a good case can be made that the experimental subjects that Pittsburgh should be using are other primates, not a man. Even if it is true that the fellow who got the baboon liver had little or no chance of getting a human cadaver liver, this would not justify using him as an experimental subject. Hopeless terminal illness is not enough of a reason to justify an experiment.

Researchers need to have adequate scientific information to support the idea that a baboon transplant might work. The best way to get this information is to do the basic work on primate to primate transplants. It is not clear that the first liver xenograft had been preceded by adequate research in animals.

There is another moral problem with the use of a baboon as the source of a liver. There are not all that many baboons around who live in healthy, disease-free environments. While the researchers at Pittsburgh clearly hope that other people might be able to benefit from a baboon transplant if the experiment works, the reality is that there are so few baboons now living in breeding colonies that it would take years, if not decades, to breed a larger number of others.

The experts at the meeting in Strasbourg agreed that over the next five years it would be very hard to find more than a couple of hundred baboons to use as possible sources of livers and other organs. If xenografting research is going to solve the terrible shortage of hearts, livers, kidneys and other organs and tissues available for transplant to those in need, it is going to have to focus on abundant animals such as pigs, cows or goats.

If the goal of transplanting a baboon liver is to find alternative sources for the thousands of people who die each year for want of organs, then it is doubtful that baboon transplants are going to be of much help even if the current experiment works. If that is so then the morality of the current experiment is less self-evident.

What Parent Wouldn't Donate?

A few years ago, a transplant team at the University of Chicago undertook a pioneering surgical experiment. Three-year-old Alyssa Smith became the first American to receive a lobe of a liver from a living donor: her own mother. All previous liver transplants for children in the United States have used organs from people who had died.

While there are acute shortages of organs and tissues for all those needing transplants, the donor situation is especially dire for young children dying of liver failure. Unlike adults, very young children do not ride motorcycles without helmets, drive cars without seat belts or shoot each other in the head.

There are about 700 children in the United States who are diagnosed each year as needing a liver transplant. Roughly a third of them die while waiting for a donor organ. The Chicago transplant team decided to try the live-donor approach as a way to get around the shortage of cadaver organ donors.

The Chicago group commendably had given the matter of informed consent a great deal of thought. They were so concerned about the ability of the worried parental donor to give informed consent that they decided to undertake the first transplant on a child who, while suffering from liver failure, was still, relatively speaking, in good health.

The ethics of experimentation normally requires those doing experiments to take the sickest subjects first. By trying the newest procedures on those who are dying, there can be little doubt that the doctor has not made the patient worse off than he or she would have been had nothing been done. But in this case, rather than wait until Alyssa was at death's door, the surgeons decided to operate before her own liver completely shut down.

By operating before a crisis forced a quick decision, the surgeons gave Alyssa's mother more time to think about whether she really wanted to face the high risk involved in the complex, dangerous surgery necessary to remove a liver segment. But, by deciding to operate on Alyssa sooner, the surgeons also reduced the time they would have had to find a cadaver liver donor. Moreover, it is debatable whether the decision to operate while Alyssa was not in any immediate danger of dying really allowed her mother to make a more informed choice about donation.

The problem with donation between a parent and child is that it is asking an awful lot to expect a mother or father to make an "informed" choice about undergoing risky surgery when their own child's life hangs in the balance. Does anyone really think parents can say no when the option is certain death for their own son or daughter? And is the situation any different whether the mom or dad has days or months to make a choice?

Informed consent sounds good in theory, but sometimes in practice it does not amount to a hill of beans. The vast majority of parents would do anything to save the lives of their children—up to and including killing themselves. Consent does not mean much when risk assessment goes out the window.

Since parents almost always will agree to be donors for their children, basing their decisions on emotions rather than weighing the risks and the talents of the surgeons, the surgical team performing the operation had better b sure they can do it right.

It will not suffice to say that a live liver donation was done at the request of a parent. A parent's consent to risky surgery to try to save his or her own child's life is not a consent that can be trusted. The only thing that can be trusted is the scientific skill and preparation of the transplant team that offers the option of live donation.

The transplant group in Chicago had impeccable scientific and clinical qualifications. What transplant physicians and those who regulate the transplant field must now do is to insist that any other transplant team that does future live liver donations has the qualifications and expertise to do so.

Trust that the surgeons have a reasonable chance of succeeding is all parents can have when asked to risk death in order that their children might live.

Drug: If Known Risks Outweigh Uncertain
Benefits, End Study

How dangerous does an experiment have to be before you lose the right to choose to participate in it? That is the question facing the 11,000 women who are currently subjects in a path-breaking national study to see whether a drug, tamoxifen, can prevent breast cancer.

When these women were initially approached about participating in the drug study, they were told that, while there were risks associated with tamoxifen, including uterine cancer, there were no known deaths associated with the drug.

But, now, a team of University of Pittsburgh scientists overseeing the trial has issued an unusual update to the informed consent form given to all the women in the experiment. The update said new evidence from another study showed that deaths from cancer of the uterus had been caused by tamoxifen.

The thousands of women now in the study and the thousands more yet to be recruited now must decide if the possibility of preventing breast cancer is worth the real risk of developing a fatal form of cancer of the uterus.

The researchers and doctors at dozens of medical centers around the country who are still asking women to participate in the prevention study must now decide if the small but certain risk of giving a drug known to cause a fatal form of cancer to healthy women is outweighed by the benefit of learning whether that same drug might help some women at risk of breast cancer.

In April 1992, the National Cancer Institute, after much public debate and controversy allocated $68 million for this first-of-its-kind experiment. All previous research on cancer involves using new drugs or other techniques to try to kill cancer cells in people who have the disease. The goal of the Breast Cancer Prevention Trial is to see whether powerful drugs can prevent breast cancer in healthy women.

The researchers asked doctors all around the United States to offer the chance to participate in the study to women believed to be at risk of developing breast cancer. Ultimately, 16,000 women are to be recruited. Half will get tamoxifen and half a placebo.

The former study director, Dr. Bernard Fisher, was a surgeon who was a world renowned expert on breast cancer at the University of Pittsburgh. Fisher and his colleagues knew for many years that tamoxifen helps cure some women who have breast cancer. Since 1981, they followed women with breast cancer to see how many tamoxifen helps. It is through this study that they learned that tamoxifen can also be the cause of other cancers.

But exactly how many deaths are due to tamoxifen-caused cancers remains unknown. The data from the long-term follow-up of women who already have breast cancer has not yet been published.

According to a story in *Science* magazine, neither the National Cancer Institute nor the Pittsburgh group will discuss the exact details of what they know about the dangerous side-effects of tamoxifen because the data is in a paper that is being reviewed for possible publication in a medical journal.

Some 46,000 women die each year of breast cancer. Medicine's ability to cure the disease using current techniques has not really improved much during the past few decades. Therefore, it is understandable why the National Cancer Institute and scientific researchers are so eager to offer women some means of preventing it.

But simply telling women that they can choose between the risk of one form of cancer and another is a miserable choice. To even offer such a dilemma requires that whatever information is available about the risks of tamoxifen be made available immediately to the study subjects and their doctors.

It is also important that the scientists who are carrying the two-edged sword that is tamoxifen must be ready to shut their study down if they know that the risks of participation are more certain than the benefits.

Doctor's Fabrication of Results Hurt
Key Breast Cancer Study

Dr. Roger Poisson of St. Luc's Hospital in Montreal may well go down in history as guilty of one of the most serious breaches of the ethics of human experimentation.

On March 13, 1994, John Crewdson of the *Chicago Tribune* revealed that Dr. Poisson, the former director of the cancer center at St. Luc's, had, for more than a decade, submitted false and inaccurate data in the single most important study every conducted of breast cancer. Federal investigators say that from 1975-1991 he falsified data on at least 100 of the 1,511 patients he involved in the study.

The study, the National Surgical Adjuvant Breast and Bowel Project, sponsored by the National Cancer Institute and the American Cancer Society, is the most important source of information about breast cancer. Data on thousands of women with breast cancer, from the time of their diagnosis through various forms of treatment, has been collected from nearly 500 medical centers from all over North America.

The study is quite simply the gold standard for evaluating the effectiveness of treatments for breast cancer. Most of what is known about the prospects of success with surgery, chemotherapy and drugs such as Tamoxifin is based on this study. The recommendation that women with some forms of cancer of the breast need not undergo total removal of the breast but can do equally well with a lumpectomy, a much less mutilating form of surgery, is based almost entirely on a 1985 report of the study's findings. An ongoing experiment using the drug Tamoxifen to try and prevent breast cancer even though it is known to cause uterine cancer and other problems is based on the data in the study.

Dr. Poisson, by his fraud, has left hundreds of thousands of women with a dread disease less certain about their treatment. By his actions, Poisson has turned the gold standard into a baser metal.

Poisson's fraud in so important a study raises a number of ethical questions that administrators at St. Luc's, the National Cancer Institute, the study directors and the American Cancer Society must answer.

How was it that Dr. Poisson, who contributed results on 15 percent of the subjects in the breast cancer study, was able to keep his deceit going for so many years without being detected? What sorts of measures were taken to audit the data being turned in from the hundreds of hospitals in the study to pick up errors or outright fraud? How did Poisson manage to pull off his fraud right under the noses of his peers and colleagues for so long a time? And why, having jeopardized a study so crucial to the health of women all around the world, is Dr. Poisson still working at St. Luc's.

Why didn't the National Cancer Institute, the study directors or officials at the National Institutes of Health reveal that for more than a year they suspected that Poisson's data were flawed? Even now there has not been a paper published in the scientific literature reanalyzing the breast cancer data without Poisson's findings. Trust in the findings of the study is based solely on the word of the study directors and National Cancer Institute officials that the breast cancer study is still OK.

Why did Poisson do it? He told federal officials that he cut corners and filed false reports because he wanted to help women with breast cancer get into the study. Tragically, in his zeal to see the study progress and his own reputation grow, Dr. Poisson not only betrayed the trust of the thousands of women in the study and their doctors but also left government and hospital officials with a lot of questions to answer about how he was able to do so.

Conflicts of Interest Plague
U.S. Biomedical Research

It is beyond dispute that America leads the world in biomedical research. As President Clinton tries to restructure an economy built on 19th and 20th century products to meet the demands of the next century, American pre-eminence in biomedicine holds out the best hope of serving as the engine capable of driving that economy.

That is why every American ought to be deeply concerned about the cancer that is quietly weakening the foundations of biomedical research—conflict of interest. Recent events at the University of Minnesota's medical school illustrate just how serious the problem of conflict of interest has become and just how ineptly government, universities and legislators are dealing with it.

On February 18, 1993, University of Minnesota President Nils Hasslemo asked for and received the resignation of Dr. John Najarian as the chairman of the department of surgery.

Najarian, a doctor of international renown both for building one of the premier surgery programs in the nation and for his pathbreaking research in the field of organ transplantation, was forced to quit the job he had held for 25 years. His colleagues, peers and students were aghast that a physician of his achievement and reputation was summarily stripped of his leadership role.

The reason given for the forced resignation was that Najarian had presided over two decades of administrative mismanagement of a program run through his department to manufacture a widely used drug, ALG. ALG helps stop organs from being rejected by recipients.

There is no doubt that ALG works. There is also no doubt that it never got the requisite approval from the FDA required for new drugs and that ALG generated tens of millions of dollars in revenue.

Minnesota's surgery department went into the ALG business back in the 1970s because no commercial company was willing to gamble on the drug. ALG turned out to work so well that by 1986 the university approved the construction of a building on university property to manufacture and distribute it around the world.

The FDA, which was aware of the evolving success of ALG through the papers about the drug that were published in many medical journals, pushed the surgery department to obtain approval for ALG. But Najarian and his associates, knowing that the entire field of transplantation was convinced the drug saved lives, and that the drug was a minor sideline to the main activities of the department, did not fulfill the paperwork requirements necessary for FDA approval.

ALG became a problem for Najarian, the university administration and the federal government when sources in the surgery department began to leak allegations to the media about possible mismanagement of the ALG program.

Readers had to wipe away the drool from front page stories frothing with glee at the prospect of landing a fish as big as Najarian in the net of scandal. The steady drumbeat of allegations in the press caused the FDA and university officials to bestir themselves. Eventually, the president put Najarian's head on the block and the FDA halted the manufacture of ALG.

The net outcome of this mess is that one of the few surgeons in the world who actually believed in the importance of clinical research is out of a chairmanship and patients are at risk of dying because they cannot get a drug that works.

What is distinctive about the ALG case at the University of Minnesota is that it is not. Conflicts over what to do when money, commerce and academia mix are being played out in dozens of universities around the United States.

At one school a researcher holds back on negative findings he has on a drug until he can dump the stock he owns in the company that makes it. At another, university doctors begin routinely using a new test to identify early signs of cancer without telling patients or their community doctors that the test has never been approved by the FDA or that they hold patents on it and stand to make a fortune if it is widely adopted.

Relationships between industry and universities are proceeding in an ethical vacuum. There are no federal policies, and university policies—when they exist at all— vary widely from school to school. Administrators and lawyers are familiar with the policies; researchers are not.

If the alliance between business and the academy in biomedicine is to be the motor driving America's economy in the years to come, then someone had better get busy now writing the rules for traveling along this new road.

CHAPTER 10
VIRTUE AND VICE IN BIOMEDICAL SCIENCE

Rats! We're Going to Be
Fed More Diet Data

Roderick T. Bronson, a researcher at the Tufts University School of Veterinary Medicine, is using government money—your tax dollars—to support a cruel experiment that can only produce a result that will make your life miserable.

Yet, no congressional inquiries are being launched. No protests bubble up from the bureaucratic bog that festers inside the Washington Beltway. The President has said nary a word about this university scandal. It is left to me, your humble servant and friend, to sound the alarm, lest malevolent science wreak havoc upon you and yours.

The innocent helpless victims of Dr. Bronson's fiendish, misanthropic "research" are mice and rats. Bronson has cruelly subjected 1,400 of these cute rodents, kin to Mickey, Minnie and Mighty, to reduced-calorie diets. They have, according to a press release issued by the agency complicit in this despicable madness, the National Institute on Aging, coerced our furry little friends into getting by on a diet consisting of 40 percent fewer calories than they would normally eat. And this cruelty, this deprivation of helpless, defenseless fellow mammals has been allowed to go on *for the entire life of these creatures*!

Now you know. Bronson has been putting hapless mice and rats on a forced diet at government expense. You say you care not a whit about what rats get to eat? You say you don't see why a mouse should be spared the kind of experience Tommy Lasorda or Kathie Lee Gifford babble about incessantly in extolling the virtues of your drinking a watery, colloidal milkshake twice a day? You say you feel safe sprawled on your sofa, conducting your own research as to precisely how many carbohydrates can be ingested during four quarters of football or one 30-minute soap opera? Pay attention, bubba. Dr. Bronson is coming to get you.

See, the little critters who were put on the low-calorie diet wound up living 29 percent longer than those Bronson allowed to eat as they wished. By the time half the rats and mice on the forced "fast" had died of old age, all of the buck-toothed gnawers on the eat-all-you-can plan had long since gone to the Big Mousetrap in the sky. Not only did the dieting rodents live longer, they did not get as sick as their gluttonous peers.

Fifty-one percent of the chubby females got tumors after 24 months; only 17 percent of their slimmer sisters were stricken. The rates for meaty murine males were worse: all the tubbies got tumors, but only 17 percent of the more slender models did.

Bronson and his sponsors include the usual scientific cautions in their recent report on this so-called experiment. You can't infer much about humans from rats, the physiology of mice is poorly understood, more study is needed ... blah, blah, blah.

Forget it. The handwriting is on the wall. What's good for mice and rats will soon be recommended for you. You have been warned. Let your congressmen know where you stand. They probably have bounced enough checks stuffing themselves at fancy restaurants to know where you're coming from.

Donors Don't Need to Give Up Privacy, Too

In May of 1991, the media went loopy over the revelation that three fatal cases of AIDS resulted from organ transplants.

Front-page headlines and top-of-the-broadcast TV accounts screeched that a single cadaver donor that turned out to have been HIV positive was the source of organs and tissues given to more than 50 people.

The media wanted medical experts to provide reassurance that the transmission of AIDS in this case was a rare fluke. But no such assurance can be provided, not in an era when more than 100,000 Americans have died from AIDS, and tests for the AIDS virus are not perfect.

Frustrated by the realization that nothing can be done to totally eliminate the risk of AIDS transmission from transplants, media attention shifted to the donor's identity. Who was the person who had harmed rather than helped others by making the gift of life? The media dug hard and, a few days after the story of the fatal AIDS transmissions by transplants broke, an Atlanta newspaper got the answer.

The Associated Press, CNN and *The New York Times* were among others willing to name the source of the AIDS transmission, a 22-year-old Virginia man shot to death by a robber in 1985 while working at a gas station.

When the subject is rape, prostitution or a possible rape/sex scandal at the Kennedy estate in Palm Beach, Fla., the press flagellates itself in moral fervor about the ethics of disclosing the names of those who might have been involved. But, when the subject is medical, media people don't appear to feel any hesitation about making the name of an HIV-infected person known from coast to coast.

They should. When the press discloses the names of organ and tissue donors, it is putting lives at risk. If families refuse to consider organ and tissue donation because they fear the loss of their own or their loved one's privacy, if they turn aside a request to consider donation because they do not want to risk having some unknown dirty laundry discovered and aired in public, then some who need hearts, livers, heart valves and lungs may die for lack of donors.

The mother of the Virginia donor told reporters that her son "tried to do something for other people, and look how it turned out."

What will happen to those waiting for their chance at lifesaving transplants if the relatives of those who die fear that their altruistic act may turn into recrimination and finger-pointing on network television?

What will happen to the supply of cadaver organs and tissues if you and I begin to wonder if consenting to cadaver donation is consenting to have the most intimate details of our loved one's lives examined and disclosed on radio, television or the newspaper?

The transmission of AIDS by transplantation is news. Publicly identifying cadaver donors and their families is not. Far more dangerous than AIDS for those who await transplants is a lack of respect for the privacy of donors and their families and indifference to the fragile foundation of confidentiality upon which organ and tissue donation rests.

Scientist Deserved to Be Fired

Forrest M. Mims III became unemployed in 1990. Yes, it's true, a lot of people get pink slips. But Mims' case was different. He got canned because of his religious beliefs.

I think Mims deserved to be fired. *Scientific American*, the nation's largest popular science magazine, had been looking for someone to write its "Amateur Scientist" column. This monthly feature is aimed at folks who, having failed to blow themselves into the hereafter by monkeying around with do-it-yourself home-science experiments as children, are keen to continue the effort as adults.

Mims applied for the job by submitting some sample columns. The editors at *Scientific American* liked them, and he was hired as a contributor. Shortly thereafter, they found out that Mims is a fundamentalist Christian who does not subscribe to the theory of evolution. The mortified editors changed their minds.

Mims has not gone quietly. In fact, he has gone so far as to complain to the Committee on Freedom and Responsibility of the prestigious American Association for the Advancement of Science about his dismissal.

On October 29, 1990, the chairman of the committee sent Mims a letter saying that, while the committee did not want to take a stand on his firing, it believes "a person's ... religious ... affiliations should not serve as criteria in the evaluation of articles submitted for publication."

Is the major science organization in the United States saying that in firing Mims *Scientific American* is guilty of religious discrimination?

I hope not.

I believe Mims is not qualified to write a regular column about science for the general public. Would he be willing to present do-it-yourself experiments that lend weight to the theory of evolution? Can someone who is responsible for presenting science to the general public write credibly about geology, molecular biology, anatomy, genetics, ecology, ornithology or paleontology—all fields that presuppose the fact of evolution? I don't think so.

Readers who buy a magazine with "science" in its title rightly expect to read about *all* sciences, not just those that a columnist believes are consistent with his religious beliefs.

Mims claims that he is a victim of discrimination. And he is. Science magazines have the right to discriminate between potential staff members who are willing to analyze any and all claims concerning scientific truth and those who are not.

Alzado's Story About Steroids Sad But Not True

Lyle Alzado, a 42-year-old former football star, had brain cancer. That was sad. Lyle Alzado was omnipresent in the media, blaming 20 years of steroid use for the cancer that grew in his brain. That was silly.

Why did so many of us paying such rapt attention to Alzado's theories about cancer? Something about the guy apparently strikes a chord in a lot of Americans, particularly men from 20 to 50 years old. The chord does not make a pretty sound.

Alzado was a standout defensive tackle during the '70s and '80s for the Cleveland Browns, Denver Broncos and Los Angeles Raiders. As a member of the Raiders, he stuck out as a tough guy on a team that prided itself on having the meanest players in football.

Alzado was not a nice guy. He played dirty on the field. He behaved like an idiot off it. He spent a great many hours chasing down those who looked at him the wrong way and pounding them into a more respectful demeanor. He mistreated and abused his wife.

Part of the reason for Alzado's lunacy on and off the field was that he was taking large amounts of steroids. Steroids are known to increase aggressiveness and lead to mood swings.

Almost every football fan older than 10 knew that Alzado, like many other linemen in the NFL, was using steroids. So did his coaches, trainers, team owners and the NFL commissioner. They had to know, either by looking at the size of men like Alzado, or because ex-NFL athletes were more than willing to tell anyone who asked. But no one cared because the image that the NFL wanted to sell was one of size, strength, violence and power.

Lyle Alzado was the epitome of the NFL's marketing image of manliness: mean, big and tough. I bought that image, and so did millions of other football fans. But not without guilt. We all knew that guys like Alzado were taking health risks to create that image.

Many of us are willing to believe that his cancer was a form of retribution for the life he led. The problem with that is there's no evidence that steroids cause brain cancer. No cancer expert I have talked to believes that steroid abuse is a cause of brain cancer—liver problems and infertility, yes; a malignant brain tumor, no.

If that is so, then why listen to Alzado's opinions on the cause of his cancer? My hunch is that Alzado's tragedy serves other needs.

For one, we desperately want to persuade young Americans to stay away from drugs. For another, some men feel bad about indulging their fantasies of masculinity on Sunday afternoons and Monday nights by making heroes out of people who behaved like Alzado.

But kids won't stop abusing drugs because we tell them horror stories that are not true. And men will not arrive at a more enlightened view of masculinity by accepting the idea that God or fate punishes those who act like Lyle Alzado.

Even if he wanted to see it that way, Alzado's life was not a morality play. Give him credit for what he did best: knocking offensive guards on their butts and sacking quarterbacks. Let's not turn him into something he was not.